Bernard M. Patten, MD
AB, 1962 Columbia College, Summa Cum Laude
MD, 1966, College of Physicians and Surgeons, Columbia University
Fellow of the American College of Physicians
Fellow of the Royal Society of Medicine
Fellow of the Texas Neurological Society
Fellow of the American Academy of Neurology
Memory Fellow of the New York Academy of Medicine
Diplomate of the American Board of Psychiatry and Neurology

THE GREAT AMERICAN MEDICAL SHOW

THE GOOD, THE NOT-SO-GOOD, THE BAD, AND THE UGLY

• • •

BERNARD M. PATTEN, MD

THE GREAT AMERICAN MEDICAL SHOW
THE GOOD, THE NOT-SO-GOOD, THE BAD, AND THE UGLY

For permission requests, write to the publisher at:
contact@identitypublications.com.

Ordering Information:
Quantity sales. Special discounts are available on quantity purchases by corporations, associations, and others. For details, contact the publisher at the address above.

Orders by U.S. trade bookstores and wholesalers.
Please contact Identity Publications:

Tel: (805) 259-3724 or visit www.IdentityPublications.com.

ISBN-13: 978-1-969995-01-9 (paperback)
ISBN-13: 978-1-969995-02-6 (hardcover)

First Edition
Publishing by Identity Publications.
www.IdentityPublications.com

"The only good histories are those that have been written by the persons themselves who commanded in the affairs whereof they write."

— Michel de Montaigne

TABLE OF CONTENTS

PREFACE

◆ ◆ ◆

Seneca: "Ab honesto virum bonum nihil deterret."
Latin: Nothing deters a good man from doing good.

My desire is to tell you of my experiences as a patient and as a doctor. I have been a patient for 83 years and a doctor for 58. My hope is that my encounters with the medical system will help you better navigate the complexities of the present health care system, help you understand it better, and help you do better with it than I did. Can we speak frankly? The current medical system in America is a mess. Some of the doctors are not as intelligent or as knowledgeable as they were in my day. Others are excellent and quite personal. Hospitals vary in quality and performance, and medical insurance is a gigantic modern problem that needs to be fixed.

Authors have a choice. They can write platitudes and offend no one. Or they can write the truth. Truth can hurt and I hope it will hurt those who are responsible for the current mess.

Cervantes: "La experiencia es la madre de la Ciencia."
Spanish: Experience is the mother of knowledge.

Yes, experience is a great teacher. All of the experiences and the people presented here in this book are true. There are no made-up and no composite characters, and no events that didn't happen. With the current era of lies, falsehoods, bullshit, delusions, propaganda, clickbait headlines, deep fakes, pseudoscience, rumors, hyperpartisanism, misinformation and disinformation, I believe we all must stick to the exact truth and nothing but the truth.

<u>For truth is the road to wisdom and gives a great deal to think about.</u>

Jesus said, 'You shall know the truth and the truth shall make you free." He was right. Truth in hand, you might be better able to judge for yourself what is good, what is not so good, what is bad, and what is ugly about current health care in America. Knowledge is power, and I hope it will help you and yours control things to your advantage.

The Present Problem

Unfortunately, there are many brands of profitable quackery around, all of which talk of healing. Some of this is from charlatans, Hindu mystics, and other humbugs, but much of it, you will see and I will prove, is from recognized and currently highly regarded institutions and hospitals. Large sums of money can be made and are being made by misleading and exploiting the sick and anxious. Large sums of money are being made by over-treating and over-testing and (God help us) over-charging. Facility fees are the latest outrageous gimmick to suck money from the public. All these things are, in my view, economic crimes, for which nobody has been, by actual design, held to account.

Also, medical hucksterism is alive and thriving in modern America. Don't believe me? Look around you. It is there. The promise of health and longevity is often the open sesame to the sucker's purse.

The United States government does not have the power or the legal tools to defend you and your family from health huckstering. You have to do it yourself. You have to identify and shun the easy and stupid entreaties that these frauds use to rope you in and get your money. Be an informed skeptic when it comes to health. Please!

The abuses thrive on an incredible scale. Look at YouTube. There you will hear absurd nonsense. For example: "Did you know that your ears have nothing whatever to do with hearing loss?" There usually follows a reference to some famous place like the Mayo Clinic or Heidelberg University, where a scientist, after many years of research, discovered a fast and easy way to correct hearing loss. Of course, audiologists and your doctor and otolaryngologists don't want you to know about this miraculous cure, which is fast, easy, painless and requires nothing but drinking a glass of hot water at night into which has been dissolved a teaspoon of RX-P29 HEARAID, available to you by mail order, for a price, for a price.

Please do not be duped by those billboard ads and magazine ads, and YouTube videos that promise the moon but usually deliver nothing much. Don't throw your money away. Beware! Be critical! And be careful! Your life and your fortune may depend on it.

How Come the Mess?

The techniques of advertising and mass communication have far outstripped the regulatory and punitive powers of government. That is not an accident. It is by design. Every segment of the commercial world has a powerful lobby in Washington. The only one who does not have a paid lobbyist is you, and your people—you and yours are at the end of the line.

Try to remember your hospital is not your friend, and it isn't your enemy either. It is a business and out for a profit. Scary! Your health insurance company is not your friend, either, and is not your enemy. But these two mammoth organizations can become contentious and even move into adversarial modes. If that happens, remember you are an amateur against a phalanx of professionals. Sorry to tell you that, under some circumstances, you will need to get a lawyer to even the odds and level the playing field.

Getting a lawyer might be hard if the amount of money involved in your claim is small. In that case, be your own lawyer. You can do this by lawyering up. YouTube videos are available to instruct you. I have done this many times, suing Blue Cross and Blue Shield, suing the Galveston Appraisal District, suing a trucking corporation for a broken windshield, suing Medicare for saying an MRI on my patient wasn't necessary, and so forth. All cases were decided in my favor.

In fact, when small amounts of money are involved, the companies would rather settle in most cases to avoid paying legal fees. When you are a lawyer, you don't have to worry about paying your lawyer $500 an hour. They do.

About This Book

This book is organized into two parts. Part One from the past, what some physicians (myself included) consider the golden age of medicine, and Part Two, which discusses my personal experiences with modern medical care, both as a practicing doctor (Section A) and as a patient (Section B). In between part one and part two, you have an intermission in which we relax and I expose for your amusement and serious consideration some great medical faux pas. Those who don't remember the past are doomed to repeat it.

After the intermission, I will frankly discuss the claims game played by medical insurance companies. Sorry to tell you the truth: You are insured until you get sick. Then you often must work hard to collect. Sorry to tell you the truth: Your health insurance company is not out there to pay for your medical care. No way!

<u>The main focus of your health insurance company is to make profits and the way they do that sometimes is by systematically delaying payment, lowering payment, and/or denying claims. The denials are not occasional or accidental but the result of a systemic focus on increasing profits by tapping a new source of revenue that comes directly out of the pockets of their most vulnerable customers, namely you.</u>

The recent Senate investigation showed multiple denials of health care for older people with stroke and falls. United Healthcare led the pack in percentage of denials with 22.7% denials. The denials helped United Healthcare take in a ton of money. UnitedHealthcare is the ninth-largest company in the world and the largest health insurance company by revenue. On December 20, 2024, its total market value was $460.3 billion, with an annual revenue of $371.6 billion, with last year's income (according to WIKI) at $32.4 billion. STOP! Think of all the health care and medical research that kind of money could have bought. Think of all the health benefits not paid. Think of all the lost health to humanity.

When push comes to shove, insurance companies defend their actions in phony, complicated, byzantine appeal procedures and, if that does not work, lots of riga-marole in court generated by their battalions of attorneys. They will often (falsely, I believe) claim their denial of claims is an attempt to improve medical care and reduce the cost for everyone. That is nonsense on stilts. If you look at the movie *Rainman*, you will hear the insurance company, Great Benefits, explain that ra-tionale to the jury. The jury recognized nonsense when they heard it and came in with a $50 million award to the estate of the kid now dead.

The real reason for the denial is (often) to line their pockets with money. If you don't think this is a problem. Think again. You are in the minority. A Gallup poll released December 6, 2024, found that Americans believe health care quality is at a 24-year low. Those polled said health care coverage is even worse, with the majority saying it is fair or poor. Eighty percent of the 1,001 adults interviewed said the cost of medical care was too high. The reason the cost is too high is ex-actly that—the prices are too high, way too high. That is a tautology, but it is the truth. And the reason the costs and prices are too high is that the American public has, for too long, tolerated too high prices from for-profit health care providers. As soon as profit is involved, you can bet there will be overbilling, overcoding, cheating on time spent, bad faith, misdealing, and even fraud. A future historian looking back at the social and economic trends of our past low-down, dishonest decade might be struck by how thoroughly dysfunctional the health care system of the most powerful nation on Earth has become.

Thus, you might sum up this book as a reading and a discussion of medical realities and philosophy, past and present, plus a consumer's guide, all informed and colored by true stories, whose purpose is designed to help you survive the system.

This is simply a book I had to write. I had no choice. Writing became a magnificent obsession. And it was only after it was written that I realized what it meant.

Fighting health insurance companies for myself and for my patients has been my part-time job for decades. If you want to know how widespread the problems are, just bring up the subject at the next party. Everyone will have a story to tell. Horror stories abound on YouTube about policyholders who got sick and suffered while fighting insurance companies about important health issues. For instance, take a look at the step-up system. Many health insurance companies require you to take the less expensive (and often less effective treatment before stepping up to the better, more effective, and usually more expensive treatment. Meanwhile, some patients, while waiting to step up, will actually die. That's good for the insurance company but not so good for the insured.

The Organization of this Book

Instead of chapters, you have encounters, and I ask you, dear reader, to study each encounter and judge it. Decide in your own mind whether the encounter showed good medicine, or medicine that was not so good, or medicine that was bad, or medicine that was ugly.

You decide, the good, the not-so-good, the bad, and the ugly! Decide on the basis of facts and not conjecture. Use facts, not faith. Do not use faith as an excuse for not thinking. Do not use faith as an excuse for disregarding evidence.

Sometimes I will be unable to hold myself back, and I will give my appraisal. That's just me. What really counts is you and your appraisal. I am too old to change much of anything. But you are not. The future is in your hands for better or worse. Good luck with it! And good luck to you!

All the best wishes,
Your friend,
Bernie

ENCOUNTER ONE
I WAS BORN

ENCOUNTER ONE: I WAS BORN

◆ ◆ ◆

All the New York newspapers and the meteorological instruments agree that the day of my birth was a dark, cold day.

An unseasonable snowstorm had started late in the afternoon and, by 8:00 that evening, had become a blizzard. While the furious flakes fell slantwise against dingy street lamps, and snow drifted among the crooked crosses and tilting head-stones of nearby Calvary cemetery, on Sunday March 23, 1941, at 9:57 in the evening, I arrived from I know not where, feet first, into the delivery room of the Astoria General Hospital, in the beloved borough of Queens, home of the happy.

Blue and yellow by breach delivery, I was already in trouble with the medical system, a state that would come and go throughout the remainder of my life for both health and non-health-related reasons.

Doctor Lanza, our family physician, hoped to bring me back to life by breathing life into my airless lungs and by restarting my little heart. He succeeded, but not without paying a terrible price. The next day, he gave my grieving parents the bad news.

"He's brain-damaged beyond repair," Doctor Lanza stated. "He will never recover. Hopeless—that's what it is. Place him in a foundling home or an orphanage, or, better still, leave him here, and I will take care of everything."

I don't remember any of this, but I am reporting what my father, Bernard, and my mother, Olga, have told me about the situation. The matter was to be repeat-edly discussed at family dinners far into the future, so I think it is pretty much the truth. What was meant by the good doctor's "everything" would be the main topic of discussion.

Thinking darkly on the subject, I suppose I could have been left to die in my crib in some drear and dusty corner of the pediatric ward, unfed and dehydrated. Or perhaps one evening between nursing shifts, Doctor Lanza himself might have, with some soft downy pillow, smothered me to death. And perhaps, in his own mind, he might have considered that he would have been doing me and my fam-ily, and society a favor.

3

Who knows?

By this year (1941), the Nazis had already taken over parts of Europe and instituted a program of euthanasia of what they considered defective people, including Jews, cripples, psychotics, homosexuals, idiots, prisoners of war, Sinti, Romas, and (God help us!) brain-damaged children.

The Nazis kept excellent records, so there is no doubt this happened. If you are interested, there are complete records, which can be seen and studied, of the dates of death, names of the victims, their age, their disabilities, and so forth. These horrors have been described often enough, though less often believed. Most of the victims were not told what was what. I assume they did not want to die. Who does? Those who deny that the haywire Nazi society practiced this form of murder are fools. The serious question remains: why did they do it? We still don't know fully why this happened, and we still don't fully understand why the German people and major free world leaders let it happen.

These events do prove that under some circumstances, humans have a capacity for evil on a scale that is beyond the beyonds, impossible to understand.

We are indebted to the Second World War for enriching our knowledge of the psychopathology of the masses, but we need to know much more in order to prevent it from happening again. Every age has its own psychopathology, and every age needs its own therapy to cope. Our age is no exception. So let us be alert. Since Auschwitz, we know what evil humans are capable of, and since Hiroshima, we know what is at stake.

Come to think of it, what Doctor Lanza was proposing does look like a kind of mercy killing. No doubt such still goes on, and I know as a medical student and doctor, many patients were "let go" for various reasons, usually because their disease was considered incurable, or required too much time and work, or the doctors thought the patient had suffered enough. Recently, there has even been much administrative talk about the waste of medical facilities, with pressure on individual doctors to give up on difficult patients and let them die. Specific examples of that practice, which are current covert forms of euthanasia, are discussed and demonstrated in my book entitled *Neurology Rounds with the Maverick*. Patients who had paid into the medical insurance system for decades were thought, usually by hospital administrators, to be wasting time, energy, and (mainly corporate) money in their care. Sad to say, in my opinion, hospitals have become money-hungry corporate giants while still pretending to be the semi-eleemosynary institutions they are supposed to be. Overcharging by hospitals is a gigantic problem. Houston Methodist has charged me $1,095 for an electrocardiogram with interpretation when the average fee for that service nationwide varies between $50 and $55 (ref. Texashealthcarecosts.org)

Houston Methodist is acting like the giant corporation it really is—interested in business and getting business. It has used the techniques of social marketing, advertising, and public relations to promote its products. Thus, we have billboards proclaiming Houston Methodist is best for digestive care in Texas, has the most advanced mammography in 10+ locations, best in neurological care in Texas, leading medicine, delivering tomorrow's care today (which is logically impossible), #1 hospital in patient cancer care, best in orthopedic care, "their experts beat my cancer" and so forth. The messages appear on multiple billboards and in glossy magazines. They must cost a fortune that might have been better used to care for the sick, the needy, and to reduce the size of medical bills. Like the claims for sugarless gum (four out of five dentists recommend…) or headache medicines (the number one pain reliever…) or camel cigarettes (nine out of ten doctors smoke Camels), Houston Methodist has something to sell just like the competition Memorial Hermann, Saint Lukes Hospital, and UTMB (University of Texas Medical Branch), Mayo Clinic, Cleveland Clinic, Columbia Presbyterian Hospital, etc. Believe it or not, in the golden age of medicine, hospitals and doctors did not advertise. It was considered unethical. As an old-school physician, I still believe it is unethical for a doctor or a hospital to advertise. How about you? What's your view?

The reasons for what is going on are complex. But most of the problem revolves, I think, around the profit motive, corporate control of medicine, and, frankly, just plain greed. Hospital payment for a patient is often just a lump sum based on the diagnosis. This is the reason for the rush to discharge.

Medicare and insurance carriers (usually) have a set fixed fee. Whether you stay four hours or ten days in the hospital, it will receive the same amount of money. The faster you are out, the less it costs them.

Therefore, the pressure to maximize profits is to make the most diagnoses and to get you, the patient, out of the hospital as fast as possible.

Payment for doctors, on the other hand, often depends on time spent. That is the root cause, in my experience, of over-coding, over-billing, double-billing, mountains of charts and paperwork, and billing for services not rendered.

My view: The doctors cheat the system on time by billing for time not worked to try to make up for the insurance companies and Medicare cheating them on money. To quote my neurologist friend, Donald Palatucci, "They cheat us on money so we cheat them on time."

Some payments are contingent on and depend on the diagnosis. That has led to multiple diagnostic labels applied to a patient for even a trivial visit. For instance, my recent visit to the eye doctor for new glasses resulted in new eyeglasses and the following diagnoses: H25.13 H25.12 H16.102 H11.153 H25.042 Z96.1 H35.372 H17.812 codes that indicate nuclear cataracts, posterior subcapsular cataracts, puckering of the macula, pinguecula, keratitis, opacity of cornea, etc. none of which prevented correction of vision to 20/20 in both eyes.

Sometimes in an effort to pile on the diagnoses the wrong key is pressed and the wrong code entered. My wife Ethel was diagnosed as having cystic fibrosis, a childhood condition she never had and never will have since she doesn't have the gene for that disease. Imagine the time and effort she had to expend to correct the error. One of my social dance friends had a routine office visit, but someone somehow pressed the wrong button or sent the wrong code, and she was billed for a disease she never had. Multiple attempts to correct this over a three-month period have failed so far. The irritating thing for my social dance partner is that there have now been recent demands for payment by a collection agency and threats of a lawsuit—all of which she finds annoying since it all involves a bill for service she never got for a disease she never had. I myself have been billed over $9,000 for surgical repair of a prolapsed vagina. Since I am a man, I don't have a vagina. Since I don't have a vagina, it is impossible that I could have had a prolapsed vagina. When questioned about this error the hospital admitted the erroneous diagnosis happened and the bill was in error, but claimed it happened because my surgeon or his billing clerk, or someone else used the wrong code.

What's the problem?

For many reasons, doctors, many of them, not all, I believe right now are in a survival mode and, sadly and unethically, have no qualms about billing for extra diagnoses or for a 50-minute complex medical evaluation when all they did was wave hello and depart, spending no more than 35 seconds for a hospital visit. The old-time professionalism of physicians is out the window. Doctors or their corporate billing agents have even threatened to turn me over to a collection agent. In fact, I have been turned over to a collection agent for a trivial bill of $315, which should have been $15. The 3 in the 315 was a mistake. Correcting the error took time and multiple letters, and calls. Finally, the collecting agent apologized and admitted their client had over-billed me when the bill should have been $15, which, by the way, I had already paid. In the old days, all that would have never ever happened. The professionalism of the doctors forbade it. Doctors have lost considerable control of what they do and how they do it. Many of them are merely data entry clerks who are told by a computer program what the protocol treatment should be. My daughter tells me that insurance companies now insist on approving in advance magnetic scans and prescriptions. How the heck can the computer program know much about the hopes and needs of the individual patient? Cookbook medicine = bad medicine.

About over-billing, double-billing, over-diagnosis, over-charging, and over-testing, delayed payment, denials of payment—more later when I discuss modern medical encounters in part two.

Meanwhile, back to Doctor Lanza and Mom and Pop and the question of my survival as a hopelessly brain-damaged child.

Doctor Lanza didn't kill me or get the chance, or I wouldn't be writing this today. But Mom and Pop and I wonder what he truly meant by "taking care of everything" and if he had done it (actually killed a kid) before or after.

Bottom line: Despite the brain damage, Mom and Pop brought me home, so I owe them my life, and I owe Doctor Lanza a lot too. I really do. Not only did he save my life by restarting my heart, but he also made my life easier. Very easy and stress-free!

Those of you who have read Langston Hughes know: No one loves a genius child. The converse of this, also true, is that everybody loves a child a little crippled, a little handicapped, a little brain-damaged. And, of course, if you are brain-damaged, no one expects much from you. You don't have to get anything right, or eat your spinach at dinner, or even start, much less complete your homework. A brain-damaged kid is not expected to clean his room or learn to spell. Being brain-damaged is a cloak that protects you from any sort of demand: you have carte blanche to have fun and just be yourself. To this day, I claim this lack of discipline as the real, proximate, and only cause for my cleaning disability, my spelling disability, and my utter inability to worry much about anything.

Follow Up

The war (World War II) ended, and my brother Jim arrived the same way, breech presentation, cord around the neck, yellow and blue, heart stopped.

Doctor Lanza told Mom, "Now you have two brain damaged children. You should be ashamed. Don't have any more."

And they didn't.

And yet, and yet. Despite the authoritarian attitude of Doctor Lanza, the family loved him and probably thought, if he wished, he could walk on water. He was one of those old-time physicians from the good old days and it is probably worth examining him and his practice to see what were the pluses and minuses and to compare and contrast Doctor Lanza's medical world with what we see today.

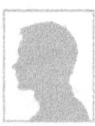

DOCTOR LANZA COMPARED TO TODAY'S DOCTORS

ENCOUNTER TWO: DOCTOR LANZA COMPARED TO TODAY'S DOCTORS

♦ ♦ ♦

"Of the several factors that contribute to wisdom, I should put first a sense of proportion: the capacity to take account of all the important factors in a problem and to attach to each its due weight."

— Bertrand Russel

Doctor Lanza was the go-to doctor for just about every serious surgical or medical thing that happened to our family. He was the first human being to touch me as he pulled me from out of my mother from the great unknown into this world. I can't recall what he looked like then. His picture in the family album shows him to be a fit man, with jet black hair and a sharp pointed nose. He was handsome in that Italian sort of way and people loved him, especially the Vaccaro's, the Italian half of the family.

Joseph V. Lanza graduated from New York Medical College in 1925. That made him 41 years old when he delivered me from death. In addition to private practice, he directed the tumor clinic at New York Polyclinic Hospital and he consulted at the Hospital for Joint Diseases, Queens General Hospital, and he consulted at the then-famous French Hospital, run by the Sisters of the Holy Cross, but now closed for lack of money. In the novel Godfather, Vito Corleone's gunshot wounds were treated in the French Hospital. In the old days, it was considered a great hospital.

Doctor Lanza's office was at 38-02 31st Avenue in Long Island City. That building is still a medical office of some sort according to Google Earth but Doctor Lanza is long gone.

At family gatherings, there were two hot and often repeated topics about Doctor Lanza. The first, but not the most talked about, was that he never, at his office at least, charged a fee. No, that is not a misprint. He never charged a fee. When we visited his office, you got medical care and no mention of money. Aunt Marie, Aunt Frances, Aunt Vera, Mom and Pop all confirm there was a small box by the exit door into which, if you felt like it, you could throw some cash. Whether it was a lot—$8.00 (Pop), or a little $2.00 (Vera and Marie) or—nothing at all (Frances). Whatever the patient voluntarily threw in was okay with the good doctor. The amazing thing is that he was able to make a living. He never got rich, but somehow or other he got along.

The fact that Doctor Lanza didn't charge a fee didn't seem to trouble anyone very much but the second item of discussion did bother people. He never married. This was a matter much talked about by Mom and Pop at the dinner table, in the car on the way to the drive-in movies or on the long trip to Uncle Joe's farm in Honesdale, Pennsylvania. The question of why not marry seemed to be very important for both my mother and father. I don't know why. But it certainly was. Perhaps it was because they believed it was not natural for a man not to have a wife. Looking back on it I still wonder why this was such an important issue, such a big deal for them, and why it bothered them so much. I am sure no one ever thought that the good doctor might be a homosexual. That kind of idea, in that era, was impossible for anyone in my family to imagine or even think about the doctor.

Finally, we got an answer.

One visit, Pop asked Doctor Lanza and was told, "Medicine is a sacred calling. Real doctors have no time for family or friends or anything but the care of their patients."

That pretty much summed it up for him. His neat statement matched with his devotion to medicine and the family tried to accept it as his vocational philosophy and the mantra of his life's work. He had a vocation as clear and as vital as any in a religious order. In fact, I read in a November 2016 article in the New England Journal of Medicine that in Lanza's era, his modus operandi was not unusual. Most of the dedicated doctors in his era did not marry and they rarely charged a fee. They were philosophical practitioners who had a fanatical devotion to their art and exercised it with enthusiasm and sagacity. They disdained, I imagine, official titles and academic honors. They were hospitable, liberal minded, paternal toward the poor, and good without believing in goodness.

Needless to say, times have changed, and doctors do marry and charge fees, and I no longer hold my boyhood belief that doctors are persons of any special importance or intelligence.

Many of the ads (and some articles) I read in the medical journals these days are about how doctors should charge, should code, should write congress for more money and less work, and how to avoid burnout and have private time and fun with friends and family. The major topic of concern seems the welfare of doctors themselves and not so much about the welfare of patients.

Don't believe me? Take a look at an ad from the New England Journal of Medicine, April 4, 2024, by Berkshire Health Systems seeking physicians. "At BHS, we also understand the importance of balancing work with quality of life. The Berkshires, a 4-season resort community, offers world-renowned music, art, theater, and museums, as well as year-round recreational activities from skiing to kayaking."

Another example, each day I get a notice from the Texas Medical Association. The notices deal a great deal with payment and how to take care of your life as a physician, how to avoid burnout, how to get lessons on proper coding for better payment, and so forth.

The American Academy of Neurology now has at its annual meetings several sessions on practice management, coding, management of insurance claims, billing, public relations, personal health, personal fitness and, believe it or not, advertising by way of self-promotion to help get referrals. In my day, all the sessions were about neurology and science and nothing but. In my day, it would have been considered a sin to spend precious meeting time on anything but science and methods to improve patient care. In my day, the Archives of Neurology had no advertisements. None! Now, I have to wade through pages and pages of ads (most about drugs) to get to the science stuff.

My generation of physicians, I believe, was more concerned with medicine itself and scientific progress than with lifestyle. But we were not as dedicated to the practice of medicine as Doctor Lanza and the doctors of Lanza's generation. But we were much more dedicated to the profession of medicine than the current crop of doctors seems to be.

Conclusion: there were giants in the earth in the old days, especially in medicine and Doctor Lanza was one of them.

OK. That was about Doctor Lanza. Now let's examine his medical practice. The past is a different country. They did things differently there. What were the pluses, and what were the minuses?

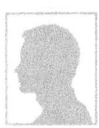

ENCOUNTER THREE

NEEDLESS SURGERY

ENCOUNTER THREE: NEEDLESS SURGERY

◆ ◆ ◆

Doctor Lanza took out my tonsils. I remember this event very clearly. He leaned over me, standing over me, appearing upside down. With his white mask covering his face like a bandit, he stared directly at me with dark, serious eyes, eyes even more piercing than his lancets. He put a cloth over my nose and mouth and said, "Breathe deeply. When you awake, you can have all the ice cream you want." Suddenly, I saw pinwheels of whirling blues, reds, greens, and yellows, and then …nothing.

When I awoke, there was blood on my pillow, and my throat was sore. A cute nurse hovered over me. "Do you want some sherbet?" It was orange, cool, and delicious.

Now, in retrospect, we know most of the tonsil operations done in that era are not needed and were done out of a sense of protocol because the medicine at the time thought, without much evidence, that such operations were necessary to prevent infections. Probably the opposite is true. Removal of tonsils probably increased the chance of infection and did not decrease the chance.

Furthermore, it is clear Dr. Lanza administered the anesthesia. It was probably chloroform or ether. The hazards of those are well known. Ministration of that anesthesia by a rag over my face was very primitive indeed. And it is likely my blood oxygen was not monitored during the operation the way, by modern standards, it would have been. Probably, I sustained some additional brain damage. Who knows?

Why was my tonsillectomy not needed? The current indications are repeated infections or obstruction of breathing or both. None of those problems did I ever have, and most kids never have severe enough obstructions or frequent enough infections to require surgical removal of the tonsils. So, tonsillectomy is going the way of bleeding or snake oil as a form of treatment.

So what!

Lesson: There are plenty of fake treatments in this world that bellow for fake charms. Watch out!

Talking about unnecessary surgery reminds me of:

Axillary Dissection for Cancer of Breast—The Bell Tolls for Thee

When I was a fourth-year medical student on surgery rotation, I was required to assist Dr. Cushman Haagensen in breast cancer surgery. The idea at the time was to remove all of the cancer and all of the breast and all of the lymph nodes and other tissue in the axillary region to prevent the spread of breast cancer. When I naively asked during an operation, "How do we know for sure that all this surgery is necessary?" Doctor Haagensen, shaking the bloody scalpel in his right hand at my face, screamed, "Leave the room immediately and never come back. I never want to see you again here or anywhere."

And that was that. I was never permitted to assist or even watch any of his operations. Some other student had to substitute for me. From then on, my job on surgery was wound care. I became very good at draining pus and curing infections. Wound care was better for me than holding retractors for Doctor Haagensen. I actually liked cleaning wounds, and the patients liked me doing it. It was wonderful watching the infections come under control and the wounds heal.

In my deep heart's core, I still think that my question about the surgery was valid. At the time, I genuinely believed that the most complete removal that was being done was right for the patient's ultimate survival. I was merely asking about what was scientifically known about the procedure and what was not known. The very defensive answer proved that much more real scientific research was needed.

Martin Arrowsmith asked Doctor Davidson, professor of Materia Medica, a similar question. "Dr. Davidson, how do we know ichthyol is good for erysipelas? Isn't it just rotten fossil fish—isn't it like the mummy-dust and puppy ear stuff they used to give in the olden days?"

"How do we know? Why, my critical young friend, because thousands of physicians have used it for years and found their patients getting better, and that's how they know and how we know!"

"But, honest, Doctor, wouldn't the patients maybe have gotten better anyway? Wasn't it maybe *post hoc, propter hoc*? Have they ever experimented on a whole slew of patients together, with controls?"

"Probably not—and until some genius like yourself, Arrowsmith, can herd together a few hundred people with exactly identical cases of erysipelas, it probably never will be tried! Meanwhile, I trust that you other gentlemen, who perhaps lack Mr. Arrowsmith's profound scientific attainments and the power to use such handy technical terms as 'control' will, merely on my feeble advice, continue to use ichthyol!"

<u>Modern Lesson: Ichthyol does not cure erysipelas or anything else.</u>

Erysipelas is a skin infection by small microscopic organisms called bacteria. Bacteria do not commit suicide, and they cannot be bluffed. Either the patient kills the bacteria with antibodies produced by the patient's own immune system and/or the bugs are killed by antibiotics like penicillin or cephalexin. In my view, it is important to kill the bacteria before they kill the patient. Ichthyol is a waste of time and bad medicine. It doesn't kill bacteria. Think of this: all that money and all the time spent on ichthyol but accomplishing nothing.

Now it looks like radical dissection for breast cancer is out of favor, and simple removal of the cancer and some X-ray treatment of the area results in just as good, if not better, results, and with far fewer side effects.

Lesson: Always ask, "How do we know for sure that this is the right thing to do?" If you do ask such a question, you will be surprised by how little is actually definitely known about a number of modern medical procedures.

<u>Much of modern medicine, believe it or not, is guesswork and a lot of it is out of joint and needs us (you and me) to set it right.</u>

One of my classmates, Dave Schuster, an otolaryngologist, gave a lecture on Tinnitus (ringing in the ears). He said, "We don't know what it is. We don't know what causes it. And we don't know what to do for it. So, let's go have a beer." That kind of honest approach applies to at least 186 diseases I can think of.

But what do you do if you don't know what to do? You can't tell the patient you don't know what to do. Who wants a doctor who doesn't know what to do? Answer: When you don't know what to do, you order a test. That's why many of the tests are a waste of time and money.

The history of medicine is littered by operations and procedures that ought not to have been done or given. Sir William Osler, who was considered the greatest clinician of the Anglo-Saxon world at the turn of the last century, taught his students that most of the drugs and other methods of treatment available to the physicians of his time were essentially useless. Yet he enjoyed an enormous reputation as a healer during his chairmanship of the Department of Medicine at Johns Hopkins Hospital in Baltimore. After he became the Regius Professor of Medicine at Oxford University, he repeatedly stated that his success as a healer was due to aspects of his personality and behavior independent of his scientific knowledge. In his 1910 article *The Faith that Heals* he said, "Our results at the Johns Hopkins Hospital were most gratifying. Faith in *Saint Johns Hopkins,* as we used to call him, an atmosphere of optimism, and cheerful nurses, worked the same sort of cures as did Aesculapius at Epidaurus."

Osler gave it for his opinion that the history of medication is the history of the placebo effect more than of intrinsically valuable and relevant drugs or operations. Aye, there's the rub. Therein lies the explanation for the puzzling fact that all ancient and primitive societies had successful healers, though medicine had little to offer, until a few decades ago, in the way of effective therapy. Ataractic drugs, the laying on of hands, Zen, supplements, energy drinks, specially treated drinking waters, meditation, biofeedback, some yoga practices, faith in a saint, a person, or a good physician are of imagination all compact in benefiting from the well documented and usually partially effective (mysterious and poorly understood) placebo effect.

Some examples of bogus treatments of a bygone era:

Bleeding was a first-line treatment for many conditions and was widely used for centuries. George Washington likely was bled to death because his pharyngeal abscess was treated with severe, extensive bleeding. Washington's doctors gave their illustrious patient what was believed to be the best treatments that orthodox eighteenth-century medicine could deliver. They blistered George's skin to draw off the fetid liquids that lurked (they thought) within. They applied poultices of wheat bran to his legs and feet. They administered calomel, mercury chloride, to empty his bowels and eliminate the toxins (they thought) were slowly killing the sunken father of America. Four times in 24 hours, they bled Washington, over the objection of Martha Washington, the concerned wife, who felt the bleeding was weakening her man. They cut a vein with a lancet and drew off 32 ounces of blood each time. All of this was strictly state-of-the-art medicine. Think of this: It was Washington's misfortune to live in an era when mercury poisoning and bleeding were at the cutting edge of health care. My opinion is that had he not received such care, Washington would have lived longer. That opinion is not just my own. Willian Cobbett wrote Doctor Rush, blaming Rush's theories for Washington's death. Cobbett said he felt "the devastating bleeding and the purging with mercury almost certainly hastened Washington's death, and it ensured the painful demise of an uncounted number of ordinary citizens as well."

In the same era, King Charles II died, probably as a result of repeated bleeding. In a single year (1827), France imported 33 million leeches after its own supplies ran out. That's how popular bleeding was in France.

Purging was a popular treatment of dubious value, and then there was a time when powdered mummies, believe it or not, had a heyday. Powdered mummies were, believe it or not, ground-up Egyptian mummies and used as medicine. As is the case in any commercial society, the great demand for mummy powder resulted in counterfeit mummy powders selling for vast sums. Mercury and arsenic, actual poisons, were standard treatments for syphilis even when the disease continued unabated. All these bogus treatments were regarded by physicians at the time as specifics backed by mainstream medical dicta. In their time, they were the standard of care. Today, we recognize that whatever effectiveness these treatments had was probably related to the power of placebos or simple misdirected faith. Today, if your doctor proposed bleeding as a treatment for a sore throat, or mercury or mummy powders, you would no doubt exit the office right away.

Wipe your hand across your mouth and laugh, but modern times are a little better. Surf YouTube and you will find foxes' lungs are good for asthma and T.B., and that ears have nothing whatever to do with hearing loss, as has been proven by a discovery from Harvard that the medical profession and hearing aid manufacturers don't want you to know about.

Today I got a message about a secret prayer that is so effective the Pope doesn't want you to know about it. The Pope has restricted the secret prayer only to his priests and bishops. How do we know the secret prayer is so effective? Here's how: The seller noticed a well-dressed man who just finished praying in the park get into his limo. Before departure, he asked the man his secret and was told "my special prayer." Of course, he didn't believe it would work, but nevertheless, he prayed the one-minute prayer every day for a week. Then, he found a lottery ticket on the ground and picked it up without thinking much about it. But presto! It won $1,000,000. So, if you want to know the secret prayer and are willing to pay a little for it, click here.

What amazes me is that some people believe this bullshit and are willing to pay for it while medical quacks, manufacturers of patent medicines and supplements, gum-chewing salesmen, and high priests of advertising live in mansions, attended by servants, and take their sacred persons abroad in limousines.

Bullshit is one of the big features of our culture. Most people know this. In my logic books, I define bullshit as something done for effect without due regard to the truth. Bullshit can be a statement or an idea or a picture, or any combination of those things. There is so much of this stuff around you must stand on your tiptoes to avoid being smothered. Bullshit is mainly harmful in the realms of advertising and public relations and the closely related realm of politics, where the bullshitter usually succeeds in getting away with something by distributing disruptive forms of nonsense. You must distinguish between what is true and what is false. Call for the facts. That is crucial, especially when it comes to medical issues.

In medicine, where most of the public doesn't understand or fully evaluate what's what, everything needs to be and should be clear, crystal clear. The diagnosis should be clear, the reason for the treatment should be clear, and the costs should be clear. Medicine needs more science, more scrutiny, and less conjecture. The most recent Journal of the American Medical Association (August 13, 2024, Vol 332, Number 6, pages 497-498) had a pointed article by Wendy Levinson, MD. Up to 30% of all tests, treatments, and procedures are unnecessary or represent low-value care, defined as care in which the harm or costs outweigh the benefits (ref: Canadian Institute for Health Information. Overuse of tests and treatments in Canada. January 12, 2024. https://www.cihi.ca). The recommendation is to reduce tests, treatments, and procedures. Daily blood tests on hospitalized patients, for example, are probably not needed for effective patient care, but do add to the bill.

Still not convinced? Consider some more examples:

In 1940, the Nobel Prize for Medicine was given to the surgeon who introduced prefrontal lobotomy for schizophrenia. The patients operated on were helped only temporarily and then they were much worse off than patients who had never been treated. If a surgeon tried to do such an operation today, he would lose his license and be drummed out of the profession. This story about how organized medicine went haywire deserves a chapter and so does the health spa business. If I am up to it, I will write about those things in the intermission. The lessons they teach are worth the effort.

Fish oil now seems to be coming back in vogue. When I was a kid, it was a fad. My mom would give me horrible-tasting cod liver oil. It is rich in vitamin D so I suppose that was the reason. Magnum doses of vitamin D were administered to arthritic patients in capsule form until some of the patients died of calcium deposits in their kidneys. Too much vitamin D is toxic and does cause kidney stones and nephrocalcinosis, the medical term for calcified kidneys.

Part of the problem is that the advice in the medical literature keeps changing. Physicians told diabetics in the old days to eat a diet high in fat because the patients had no insulin to manage the sugars. A typical diabetic breakfast tray when I was a boy in the early 1940s was eggs, bacon, lots of butter, no sugar, and very little bread. Then the profession changed its mind. The diabetic was given plenty of carbohydrates because the blood sugar elevation could be covered by insulin injections. Now, diabetics have had another change. The suggested diet resembles the normal diet: low in cholesterol and high in complex carbohydrates but easy on the simple sugars.

Diverticulitis is a common bowel condition in which small pockets in the colon become infected. Until recently, the best doctors recommended that patients with diverticulitis eat a diet low in roughage. Today, the advice is directly the opposite: Stuff in the roughage.

Cholesterol: Not long ago, there was a major misconception that the cholesterol we eat somehow causes heart disease. Eggs were singled out by the American Heart Association as causing atherosclerosis because of their high cholesterol content. That declaration was in 1968, and eggs remained in nutritional purgatory for decades, even after reams of scientific papers proved dietary cholesterol is not absorbed by humans. In humans, dietary cholesterol is excreted in the poop. The problem was that the basic original research was done on rabbits and chickens, where cholesterol is absorbed from food and deposited in blood vessels, causing atherosclerosis. Thus, cholesterol in the diet does not matter unless you are a rabbit (or a chicken). In 2015, the government finally conceded that "cholesterol is not a nutrient of concern for overconsumption." There is no connection, we now know, between cholesterol in the diet and cholesterol in the blood. None. Another health myth has been proved wrong. The vast majority of the cholesterol in your blood is produced by your liver. The amount produced and put in the blood is very much controlled by your genetic makeup and several other factors, including how much you exercise.

Treatments, like fashion, change with the wind.

When I was first in practice, estrogen, the female hormone, was used to control the symptoms of menopause. It worked, too, especially eliminating the night sweats, hot flashes and mood swings. Then, for some reason known only to God, estrogen went out of style. The idea was (without much evidence) that it just might cause breast cancer or uterine cancer. Patients had read about that in the newspapers or saw in on TV and often refused treatment and suffered accordingly. Then estrogen came back in vogue because it was thought to prevent heart disease and stroke.

Now, the main idea seems to be that estrogen might prevent osteoporosis or weak bones. In the same issue of a medical journal, I read a paper written by experts that estrogen CAUSES heart disease. Adjacent to that paper was another paper also written by experts that proved estrogen prevents heart disease. Confused? Me, too. Which is it? Could it be that in some patients, estrogens prevent heart disease, and in other patients, who might have some genetic difference, estrogens might actually cause heart disease? We doctors don't know. But it is difficult to tell a patient we don't know. Who wants a doctor who doesn't know?

The latest news (August 26, 2024) is that hormone therapy for menopausal women decreases aging and actually provides a survival advantage by delaying death. That's nice because death spoils your weekend. (reference: Liu and Chenglong—Hormone Therapy and Biological Aging in Postmenopausal Women, Journal of the American Medical Association, Netu Open 2024;7(8). Bottom line: There are still lots of unresolved questions about the use of estrogens. If you don't know what to do, analyze the situation and act accordingly.

Yet another example. When I was an assistant physician at the New York Hospital Cornell Medical Center in 1966, protocol and traditions dictated that patients who were admitted with the diagnosis of myocardial infarction (heart attack) or the diagnosis of "rule out myocardial infarction" had to be placed on complete bed rest for four to six weeks. This was standard care not only at Cornell but at Harvard and Columbia and at every mainstream major hospital and treatment center in America. The idea was to put the heart at rest so that the injured heart muscle could have a better chance to repair itself. Sitting in a chair was prohibited. Patients were not allowed to turn from side to side on their own power. If they wished to change position, they had to call the nurse to move them. The nurses also fed the patients three times a day as the exertion of feeding was considered excessive exercise that would impair healing. Going to the bathroom was also a no-no. Nurses provided bedpans as needed and moved the patients into position. Think of the inconvenience of that and the embarrassment. Think of the amount of nursing work involved.

With this treatment, the mortality was 35%, with a large number of victims dying from pneumonia or pulmonary embolism (block of lung blood vessel) from blood clots in the legs. About 67% of patients developed frozen shoulders with red, swollen left hands and arms, a condition that greatly impaired the patient's ability to dress, even when they had recovered from the heart attack.

We junior physicians were told the shoulder-hand syndrome was a reaction of the sympathetic nervous system to the heart attack. Some patients actually got their sympathetic nerves on that side cut, but without improvement. How did the professors explain the lack of improvement after sympathectomy? They said, "Well, it was just too late." Or they said, "We see it." Never was there any mention of the idea that the failure to respond to the operation meant the premise of the operation was in error, and the shoulder-hand syndrome had nothing whatever to do with the heart attack or with the sympathetic nervous system.

When some physicians proposed chair rest, not bed rest, for heart attack victims, the idea met with a storm of tremendous resistance from tradition-oriented doctors. Initial studies were not approved by the institutional review committees because chair rest was considered too dangerous. Nevertheless, some physicians went ahead (this was the era when the individual doctor had total control of his/her individual patients). Those doctors dared to get their heart attack patients out of bed and into a chair.

The results were obvious from the get-go. The patients were happier, and so were the nurses. Mortality declined to 10%. Frozen-hand-shoulder syndrome disappeared because it was due to disuse and had nothing whatever to do with the sympathetic nervous system or even with the heart attack. Pneumonia and pulmonary embolism became rare events because mobilization helped prevent stasis in the lungs, a cause of infection, and clots in the deep veins of the legs, a cause of embolism.

We now know complete bed rest is harmful for a number of reasons: it rots the bones and weakens the muscles. It causes pneumonia and pulmonary embolism. But the worst thing about it, in my view, is the mental and psychological demoralization that comes from remaining in bed 24/7.

<u>After all, in America, most of the dying takes place in a bed in a hospital, so there is a sense of safety in being out of bed. And there is a greater sense of safety in not being in a hospital at all.</u>

Although there has never been and never will be a double-blind prospective controlled study comparing bed rest with chair rest for heart attack, chair rest is now the standard of care, and bed rest is not.

The way the professors rationalized the treatment for heart attack was without merit and was draconian in extreme—the way they insisted they were right and knew the truth; the way they would brook no discussion to the contrary still troubles my sleep.

It is creepy to realize how many medical practices are not soundly based, but instead are supported by conjecture, inertia, fashion, custom, tradition, and undue respect for authority. These long-held belief systems, even when not supported by evidence, even when shown to worsen conditions, seem to become, by their recurrent use, proven treatments of value. The attitude is a tremendous impediment to progress. What modern scientific medicine needs is **MORE SCIENCE** and less guesswork.

While on my soapbox, at present, I point my finger of accusation at oncologists, who tend to intervene no matter what the costs. Usually, they are truthful about defining the small chance of benefit from their tests and treatments. If only they were as honest and forthright about the miserable consequences of chemotherapy and the costs. Better to manage the incurable diseases with common sense and compassion. When chemo was first introduced, because of the terrible side effects, I advised most of my patients to forget it and die in peace. But as the years went on, I saw some patients actually recover. But of course, only a few recovered. The lucky few. Most died of the cancer or the treatment or both. Every patient I ever referred to M.D. Andersen Hospital, the number one cancer hospital in America, died of the cancer or the complications of treatment. That is, everyone died except Herb, my best friend. He was mercifully sent home without treatment, sent home to die, which he did, in peace, a few weeks later, of pancreatic cancer, a type of cancer very hard to beat.

Sometimes it seems like the health care system is structured to torture the elderly, not because of malevolence, but because there is somewhere a (computerized?) program of a suggested protocol based on reimbursement rather than what is best for the patient. My 94-year-old mother-in-law gave it for her opinion, "Sometimes doctors do what isn't needed because Medicare will pay."

How's that for insight!

Lesson: Sometimes, the concepts we think we know so well, that have become part of us, and, automatically, part of our consciousness and belief systems, are wrong from the start. We need to change them every so often, and we need to question them always. We need to question not just general, social, economic, political, or philosophical concepts, but also, at times, the scientific and medical concepts as well. Otherwise, there will be little or no progress.

ENCOUNTER FOUR

I CURE MY OWN WARTS

ENCOUNTER FOUR: I CURE MY OWN WARTS

◆ ◆ ◆

Small semi-translucent nodules appeared on the fingers of both my hands. Mom thought it might be warts and wanted Doctor Lanza to take a look. We went to his consultation room in Long Island City. The room was at once his business office, his consultation room, his minor operating theater, and probably his living room during off hours. But never a poker den. Doctor Lanza was too busy and too dedicated to his work to play at cards.

Against the east wall of his consultation room was a cabinet of colorful medical curiosities, and beside it a full-length skeleton. "Is that a former patient?" I asked. "Nope," replied Lanza. "He's my buddy who gives me advice when I don't know what the diagnosis is or what to do."

No appointment was necessary to see Doctor Lanza, or even possible. You just arrived during office hours and sat until called by the doctor himself. There was no secretary and no receptionist, and no nurse. There were no forms to fill out. No insurance hassle. Usually, the wait time was short and there were plenty of books and magazines to amuse yourself while waiting.

Doctor Lanza greeted us by name and wanted to know how I was doing. He smiled and laughed and said he was pleased, for a brain-damaged kid, that I was doing so well. He was being humorous. We did not misconstrue the humor. By his smile, chuckle, and his body language, he showed his human face and that he really cared. Frances Peabody famously said, "The secret of care of the patient is in caring for the patient." Doctor Lanza had mastered the secret.

Doctor Lanza looked at my fingers and muttered something in Latin, which I think was the Latin name for common warts. He explained the warts were caused by a virus, and the virus had caused small skin tumors. The tumors never became malignant, so there was nothing serious to worry about. "There is no effective treatment. Most kids in a few years lose the warts. We don't know why that happens, but the warts do usually go away by themselves."

And that was that.

No record was made of the visit. What for? This whole thing was trivial. No one checked for the current coin of the realm, which is your insurance card. The whole thing lasted about eight minutes. Try to match something like that in modern times. You can't. This is not the place to discuss the real reason for the forms and for the massive consent forms that have become part of modern medicine. When someone hands you a form, they are asking you to waste part of your life. The forms are for their benefit, not yours. About forms, more later.

Pop threw eight bucks into the cash box, and we hopped back into our bright red Chrysler and headed home. The ride from Long Island City to Queens Village runs 45 minutes, so I had plenty of time to think about what happened.

Frankly, I was disappointed. After all this great dinner talk about how wonderful Doctor Lanza was, he did not deliver the cure I expected. I wanted him to lay his sacred hands on mine and have the warts disappear like magic. He didn't even write a prescription for a medicine. We left his office better informed but empty-handed. But there was a positive emotional effect from the kind way I was treated, and there was a definite hope that gave me a positive outlook on things—namely that in time there would be reasonable control over the warts, and we now knew that the warts could do no harm. They could not and would not turn into cancers.

For some unexplained reason, I felt better when I left the office. In fact, I felt much better. The visit itself actually had a salutary effect on my mentality. And I liked the doctor's quick wit about his buddy, the skeleton.

A sense of humor helps neutralize the usually solemn medical atmosphere.

I also liked the bric-a-brac and medical curiosities, and of course, the full-length skeleton. Those things gave his office a certain, je ne sais quoi, touch. Many modern offices are nearly monochromatic, lifeless, and emotionally sterile. Next time you visit your doctor's office, check it out. What pictures hang on the walls? Are there cheerful colors? Bric-a-brac? Does the place look too sterile?

Many people are afraid of doctors (me too), and the doctor showing a human trait helps abate the fright. A sense of humor is needed to help neutralize the high-tech environment of the modern hospital. Laughter is a good medicine.

Instead of a cure, what happened with my wart visit was a diagnosis and an explanation of the cause of the warts, plus a kind of prognosis. The prognosis was not exact. It was a probability statement that most kids recover.

But if most recover, then some don't. So, I didn't get absolute assurance that the warts, sometime in the future, by some unknown mechanism, would disappear. There was hope, but it was an uncertain hope. But the hope, the comfort, love, interest, hands-on touch, laughter, and confident statements about what was wrong all had therapeutic value. No question about it.

Now, in retrospect, I think this was very good medical care. It stuck to the facts. It had a special humanity.

<u>It was right in line with the ancients, who believed most human afflictions are self-limiting and cure themselves.</u>

An accurate diagnosis, arrived at through medical acumen, determines whether a particular disease is self-limiting or is potentially dangerous and therefore requires particular therapy. Good medical care can, of course, speed healing, make dealing with illness more comfortable, and perhaps make healing more complete. But in the final analysis, recovery depends on natural healing processes themselves, on the patient's own resistance to disease, and on the patient's will to live. Therein lies the explanation for the fact that all ancient and primitive societies have had successful healers, even with medicine that had little or nothing to offer and even with medicines that were harmful. The ancients were so familiar with this natural recovery process that they had a special name for it: *Vis Medicatrix Naturae*, the power of natural medicine.

The natural recovery is likely to be more long lasting. My recovery from mumps, measles, and whooping cough will protect me from reinfection for the rest of my life.

Every gardener knows the plants have this same natural tendency to recover from infection, blight, or damage from bad weather. If this process were not general throughout nature, in all the plant and animal kingdoms, life on this planet as we know it would not exist.

Talking about recovery from childhood illnesses reminds me to tell you about what happened to the warts.

While seated in the back seat of the Chrysler, I took the situation into my own hands. With my left index finger and left thumb, I pinched the wart on the index finger of my right hand and pulled the wart off. The pain was sharp and severe but lasted only a minute and the base where the wart had been bled bright red blood. I blotted the blood with my handkerchief and decided that my first operation as a surgeon was a success. I had removed a small tumor. But I decided the pain involved was not worth using the same technique on the many other warts on my fingers.

Two weeks later all the warts dried up and fell off the fingers never to return. It would be irresponsible of me to recommend this treatment. I am reluctant to write about it for fear of creating false hopes in people similarly afflicted. My cure was a case of one. Because an event follows some event it does not mean the two are related as cause and effect. The cock crows and the sun rises. That does not mean the cock caused the sun to rise. In fact, the crowing of the cock has nothing to do with the sun. The cock is just calling the hens to mate. The sun rising at the time is mere coincidence. The error in logic is called the Post Hoc Propter Hoc fallacy. But still it seems quite a coincidence that pulling off a wart subsequently was followed by the involution of all the other warts.

My case of one has small standing in the annals of modern medicine. It has little more than anecdotal or testimonial value. Modern immunology might have a theory about what happened: The warts have a mechanism that shields them from the immune system and prevents the body's recognition that they are there and that they are foreign tissue. Many cancers have such shields. By pulling the wart off its base, wart antigens (proteins? Or other tumor markers) could have been now exposed to the immune system. Now that the immune system knew the warts were there, it went to work destroying them. It is doubtful my discovery will win the Nobel Prize in Medicine, but I did enjoy writing about how I cured my own warts by the first surgery I ever did.

Evaluation time:

Doctor Lanza did a good job taking care of my wart problem. The visit was short and sweet and cheap and effective. The take away lesson is that personal touch is important in medical care and is probably the reason chiropractors and acupuncturists and physical therapists are appreciated and stay in business. Naturopathic remedies probably are partially effective due to the placebo effect and the only thing they harm is your pocket book. Trivial illnesses like the finger warts and conditions that recover by themselves are best managed by the real doctor keeping his/her hands in pockets and issuing reassurance about recovery. Securances might help relieve pain and speed recovery and possibly help insure more complete recovery. But for major illnesses that are matters of life or death or for diseases that significantly and adversely interfere with life and happiness, major treatments will be needed.

You agree?

With that idea in mind let's look at Doctor Lanza's handling of major life-threatening illnesses. Do they and does he measure up to modern expectations?

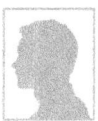

ENCOUNTER FIVE

GRANDMA ANNA DIES

ENCOUNTER FIVE: GRANDMA ANNA DIES

◆ ◆ ◆

Grandma Anna Vaccaro (my mother's mother) developed severe abdominal pain. The local doctor thought she needed an enema, but that didn't help. Her condition worsened and she was rushed to the French Hospital where Doctor Lanza did an exploratory operation opening her abdomen only to find a ruptured appendix with infectious material spread throughout the peritoneal cavity.

Ugh!

Nothing much to do about that. Doctor Lanza cleaned out what he could and packed the area with sulfa drug (one of the few antibiotics available at the time) and closed the wound. The pain was terrible and Grandma Anna died a horrible death from peritonitis, the infection in her abdomen.

Conclusion: Complete failure. We don't know for sure but it is probable that more modern imaging would have helped make an earlier diagnosis that could have been life-saving. Drainage of the peritoneal cavity might have helped with infection control and the more powerful modern antibiotics given intravenously would have helped. In the absence of certainty about what would or would not have happened we have to fall back on a reasonable probability. Modern medical care would probably have been more effective and possibly life-saving. Modern medicine certainly could not have done worse or produced a worse outcome which was a very painful horrible death for Grandma Anna. The enema was of course a no-no. It did nothing for the infected appendix and probably worsened the situation by delaying appropriate treatment. Also possible: The enema could have ruptured the appendix by increasing pressure in the gut.

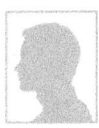

ENCOUNTER SIX

MOM GETS BREAST CANCER

ENCOUNTER SIX: MOM GETS BREAST CANCER

◆ ◆ ◆

Mom developed a lump in her left breast. She kept checking the lump every day for three months, hoping it would go away.

It didn't.

The biopsy showed invasive adenocarcinoma that looked highly malignant. Doctor Austin Johnson from Columbia surgical pathology and I reviewed the slides and actually cried together. Mom's prognosis was grim because the cancer was highly malignant, much more malignant than the usual breast cancer. There are cancers with a small c and there are cancers with a big C. Cancer is not just one disease. It is many diseases with many different types of cells with many different physiologies. The secret to curing cancer will come from a complete and detailed understanding of the physiology of each type of individual cancer cell.

Doctor Lanza did his thing—major axillary dissection with lymph node removal. The operation produced the usual pain and swelling of the arm. But the hope was that the surgery would cure the cancer.

It didn't.

Mom developed cancer that spread locally and to the brain, and probably spread to the bone. Mom became miserable with back pain.

She and Pop decided to transfer to Columbia Presbyterian Medical Center for further care because I was a medical student at the College of Physicians and Surgeons and could keep Mom company during her hospitalization. Usually, she was in Harkness Pavilion, the exclusive place for private patients. She didn't approve of the hospital food, so she always ordered a private catering service to bring me and her dinner. Those dinners were the most interesting and most intimate times I ever spent with Mom. I loved the wonderful food and conversation, and so did she. It is a rare event that, as an adult, you really get to talk to and to know your mother. I loved her then, and I still love her.

Mom felt she was dying at age 50 and she didn't like the idea one bit. Pop hated it. Me too.

Stuart Cosgriff, a world-renowned internist, volunteered to take care of Mom. That was not a misprint. He volunteered, and he repeatedly refused to accept any kind of payment. Pop begged and begged, saying, "My insurance is great. I have been paying in for decades. Please just sign the form and get paid." Doctor Cosgriff shook his head no, "Professional courtesy. I wouldn't think of charging the mother of a medical student."

Doctor Cosgriff visited Mom every day and explained what he thought. Hormone treatment was started. This was mainly testosterone. After two weeks, Mom refused the treatment. She said it was turning her into a man with a mustache, and she didn't like the fact that her behind was shrinking. "I don't want to be a man."

So, that treatment was out.

Then Mom developed total body itching. The bilirubin blood level rose, and Doctor Cosgriff thought that was the cause. The question became what to do. The cancer could be in the liver and causing the problem, or Mom could have developed some kind of liver disease like hepatitis, or there might be something else going on that we can't even imagine. Doctor Cosgriff thought there might be an obstruction that was blocking the usual exit of bile into the intestine. That was an absolutely brilliant idea. Something most people would not have thought. And so, Mom was asked to undergo an exploratory operation to check the bile drainage system. She was desperate for anything that might stop the itching, which was torturing her day and night. She consented.

Milton Porter, one of Columbia's greatest surgeons, volunteered to do the operation. That was not a misprint. He volunteered and, like Doctor Cosgriff, refused to consider any kind of payment, and like Doctor Cosgriff, he refused any payment from insurance. This was professional courtesy again. I am telling you this to prove to you that it was an entirely different era, an era where doctors were not money hungry, an era where physicians were true professionals. They were true professionals who even gave the mother of a lowly medical student professional courtesy.

Doctor Cosgriff told me and Mom he was reasonably sure, based on the distribution of conjugated and non-conjugated bilirubin, that there was an obstruction blocking the normal drainage of bile into the intestine. The way to prove or disprove that conjecture was to explore the region and directly visualize the gall bladder and bile duct.

A miracle!

At the operation, a small tumor was found blocking the drainage of bile. Doctor Porter thought it was too tricky to try to remove the tumor. The bile duct is small and delicate, and it would be risky to "annoy it." Instead, he bypassed the obstruction by sewing the top of the gall bladder to the intestine—another brilliant idea!

Bingo! Bile blood levels declined steeply, and the terrible itching disappeared. Mom became very happy until the back pain worsened.

The X-rays showed multiple lesions in the bones of the spine. Doctor Cosgriff thought this was probably the cancer. But, he said, there is a big difference between thinking you know something and actually knowing. He recommended a bone biopsy. Mom agreed.

Doctor Andrew Bassett, orthopedic surgeon, volunteered to do the bone biopsy. That is not a misprint. Andrew wouldn't even think of charging the mother of a medical student, and he never did.

The operation was done under local anesthesia, with Mom fully awake. She came out of the operating room laughing her head off. "Doctor Bassett is the funniest man alive. He had me laughing the whole time. Now, I want another bone biopsy, just to hear the jokes."

A sense of humor helps neutralize the usually solemn medical atmosphere.

Doctor Austin Johnson and I reviewed the biopsies and cried together. Under the microscope, the cancer looked very malignant. It looked very malignant because it was. No question, Mom was doomed. It was just a matter of time and tricks. I hoped Doctor Cosgriff had more tricks up his sleeve.

He did.

Doctor Cosgriff gave Mom Darvon (propoxyphene), a mild pain killer which most people would have thought inappropriate, considering we were dealing with bone cancers that caused severe pain not controlled by morphine. But another miracle! The Darvon worked, and Mom left the hospital pain-free as long as she took the Darvon every four hours. From that day forth, I became a believer in Darvon and prescribed it when appropriate.

Herb and Doris, very elderly neighbors across the street, invited us to a Christmas party. Doris met me at the door with a martini and toasted me with hers. "Doctor Bernie, you have changed my life. Because of you, my life has been wonderful for the last three years." Herb joined in toasting me with his martini, "Your medicine worked a miracle on Doris. Yes, a miracle. She went back to caring for her flowers. Flowers are her real passion. The arthritis pain completely disappears when she takes your medicine."

Then, I asked, "By the way, what was my medicine?" Together, Herb and Doris shouted, "Darvon, of course."

Evidently, my nurses have been renewing the prescription every three months for three years and doing Doris a service. Darvon is no longer available on the American market. I don't know why, but I smell a rat. Probably some other company that makes higher-powered and more expensive painkillers persuaded someone to take it off. Every medicine has side effects, and Darvon had its share, although neither Mom nor Doris noticed any. Furthermore, the instructions that come with the package insert say "no adult beverages while taking Darvon," an instruction Mom and Doris conveniently ignored.

Mom became confused and then unable to recognize me or Pop. Danny Sciarra, Professor of Neurology at Columbia, volunteered to care for her. He personally did a spinal tap and proved Mom had meningeal carcinomatosis, cancer involvement of the meninges, the soft tissue layers that cover the brain and spinal cord. Danny said he was not afraid to try an unapproved experimental medicine and would treat Mom with Decadron. Bingo! Within a day, Mom was back to her normal conscious self. She knew me and Pop and her sister Vera, and so forth. It looked like a true miracle, and in a certain sense, it was. But we all knew (Mom included) that the end was near. One night after a nice filet mignon dinner, Mom announced that she was going to die that night. I truly regret my behavior after that. I screamed at her that that was not true. "Don't talk like that." I added, "The doctors, especially Doctor Cosgriff, must have more tricks up their sleeves." Mom said, "Mickey, don't be a pest. I'm about to die, and instead of getting a little sympathy, I get yelled at."

I kissed her and left in a huff. In the hallway, just getting out of the elevator was Doctor Cosgriff himself. He pulled me over. "Sorry, I am out of ideas. The end is near. I won't be surprised if your mother dies soon, maybe even tonight."

He and Mom were right. That night, Mom died. I miss her and fight back waves of emotion when I think of my last visit with her. I feel the need to call her and apologize for my behavior. Alas, nature does not give that opportunity.

I dropped out of obstetrics and gynecology, the rotation I was on at the time, to attend the funeral and burial. Doctor Raymond Vande Wiele, the chairman of Ob-Gyn, called me in to tell me I missed a week of the rotation, so I would have to repeat the entire six-week rotation. Otherwise, he would see to it that I didn't graduate from medical school.

"You don't understand, Doctor Vande Wiele, my mother died!" He frowned, "Death in the family is no excuse to neglect your duties. You should have been here working on the wards."

I begged for mercy. No luck. He was intransigent, so I appealed to Dean Houston Merritt.

Dean Merritt was on my side, "For God's sake, the kid's mother died. Have mercy."

Eventually, the Dean and Vande reached an agreement. I would take a written exam on Ob-Gyn to be graded by a senior faculty member, not Vande Wiele, and if I passed, I would not have to do a redo. The result: B+ final grade, remission from repeat, and much resentment from Vande Wiele.

Doctor Vande Wiele proved that not every great Columbia College of Physicians and Surgeons faculty member was a nice guy. He was not nice to me and he was not nice to one of his own faculty members, Doctor Landrum Shettles, who at the time was an associate professor with tenure and a diplomate of The American Board of Obstetrics and Gynecology.

In my opinion, Landrum had more intellectual horsepower than all the other members of the faculty of Ob-Gyn put together. He certainly had more degrees, including a Master of Science from somewhere out west and an M.D. and PhD. from Johns Hopkins. His erudition was obvious from his lectures on the human ovum and D&C. The D&C lecture started by him shouting, "D&C, D&C! What would we do without D&C?" (D&C is a surgical procedure involving dilation of the cervix and curettage of the uterus lining. Curettage is a surgical scraping of the inner lining of the uterus.) A massive discussion followed of the indications, benefits, side effects, and history of D&C.

Landrum's lectures on the human egg were amazing, with the most detailed pictures of the human egg in various phases of development. Landrum was a true researcher and a pioneer in the scientific study of human reproduction. He even invented techniques on how to increase the probability of getting a male or a female child, as you please, techniques that are still in use today and explained on YouTube. Landrum was a true genius, and that may be why other faculty members, including chairman Vande Wiele, were jealous. No change that. I was there and felt the atmosphere. They were jealous, alright, but they, at least some of them, also hated Landrum. Yes, hated him. Academic medicine can be vicious. I know that for a fact. The situation came to a head in 1973.

On September 12, 1973, Doctor William Sweeney, one of the great surgeons I knew at the New York Hospital Cornell Medical Center, daringly removed eggs from Doris Del-Zio. Of course, Sweeney did not get or need permission to do that from a committee on human experiments. All he needed was Doris's consent.

Doris was unable to have children with her dentist husband John because her fallopian tubes were blocked, and the couple wanted to have a child by other means, if possible.

John took Doris' eggs by New York City taxis to Landrum Shettles at Columbia and masturbated to supply sperm for fertilization of the eggs in vitro, that is, in a test tube. Bingo! It worked! This was probably the first time in the history of mankind that a human embryo was created outside the body of a woman.

But there was a snag. Landrum and others had discovered that human embryos don't have the proper receptors to implant in the uterus until they are five or six days old. Hence, incubating the embryo in the test tube before installing it in Doris was necessary. Otherwise, without incubation, the embryo would not implant and pregnancy would not result. Ah details! See how important little details can be.

What happened next is controversial. I believe Landrum's account, and that is what I shall relate here. On day four, Chairman Raymond Vande Wiele asked to visit Landrum's laboratory and see the incubated specimen. With the tube in hand, he pulled off the plug and exposed the embryo, killing it. The sample was deliberately ruined.

Not nice. Right?

And in the American tradition the Del-Zios sued Doctor Vande Wiele and Columbia. (1978 Doris Del-Zio and John Del-Zio versus Doctor Raymond Vande Wiele and Columbia College of Physicians and Surgeons, U.S. District, Lexis 14550.)

The jury concluded that Vande and Columbia had engaged in behavior "utterly intolerable in a civilized community." Doris was awarded $50,000 in damages, and John was awarded $3. That would be about $240,000 for her and $14 for him in today's money. A month later, Landrum resigned under pressure, and he sued for damages. The result of that case is sealed, but rumor has it that Landrum got $3,000,000 and his title and laboratory back. But Landrum had had it with Columbia and founded his own clinic in New York City.

There is an interesting coda to this story. Despite many severe criticisms of in vitro fertilization, in 1983, Dr. Vande Wiele set up his own IVF clinic at Columbia. He didn't last long at it because he died of a heart attack on August 14, 1983, at age 60.

Lesson: Some medical innovations are so new that they provoke hostility, and the inventors suffer greatly. Andre Cournand was one of them. He visited the Columbia division of Belleview Hospital when I was a student there. His story pretty much matched Landrum's. Andre thought you could put a long tube in the heart and measure pressures, flow, and oxygen exactly. The human experiment committee vetoed the idea as too dangerous. So, Andre inserted a catheter into his own heart and took an X-ray of it in his heart. He proved that the catheter could be safely inserted and removed without any harm. But, of course, he lost his position immediately for violating the command of the human experiment committee. Evidently, you were not allowed, without committee permission, to experiment on yourself.

UndAunted, Andre then went to France, where he continued his work on cardiac catheterization. Columbia hired him back, and in 1954, he shared the Nobel Prize for his work. I can still see him there at Belleview smiling without rancor, seated next to the fluoroscopy room, where he experimented on himself and filmed the catheter in his heart. We six students sat in awe as he told his story. His message was clear: "Don't let the bastards grind you down."

This encounter chapter is about physicians and medicine in the old days. There were pluses and minuses. You, dear reader, can judge what was good, what was not so good, what was bad, and what was ugly. I am just trying to paint the picture and show you the facts. Next up, the case of my Great-Uncle Tom.

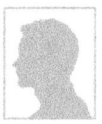

UNCLE TOM DIES

ENCOUNTER SEVEN: UNCLE TOM DIES

◆ ◆ ◆

Great-Uncle Tom lived in Astoria with my Grandma Mary, Grandpa Owen, and their children: Aunts Mary, Margaret, Agnes, Joan, and Uncles Tommy and Johnny. Sorry about all the names. I can't help it. Catholics = no birth control, and besides, Grandma Mary liked babies.

They all fit into a five-bedroom rented house one block from Steinway Street. There, while the Jewish kids went for piano lessons on Saturday, we Irish kids went for lessons in fisticuffs. And I, an Irish boy, got my lessons from Great-Uncle Tom Connors, who had been the middleweight boxing champion of the British army in Africa and who had been the Golden Gloves champion of New York City.

On Saturday, August 16, 1947, we put on the gloves as usual, and Uncle Tom told me to "put 'em up. Box!"

I can't remember if I put them up or not. Or what happened. But I know he hit me so hard, I flew against the opposite wall and collapsed to the floor.

"Uncle Tom, why did you hit me so hard?"

"You let your guard down. Never forget that lesson."

"What lesson?"

"Never let your guard down. Always protect yourself. That's the first rule. Remember. Never let your guard down. Now you won't ever forget it."

I haven't forgotten.

About four hours after the fisticuff lesson, Great-Uncle Tom fell backwards down the cellar stairs. It was afternoon, so I don't think he was drunk. But in an Irish household in that era, that was possible. There was whiskey in the living room and dining room, and a seltzer bottle too. No one thought much about just mixing themselves a drink. That is why the stuff was there.

Aunt Joan, who was in the ground-floor bedroom, heard the fall and ran to find Uncle Tom in bad shape and unconscious, face up at the bottom of the cellar stairs. Joan let out a harrowing scream, and I came running.

It was like some grade B horror movie. Terrible really. Unlike the black and white movies of the time, this was in full color. Tom's skull was broken open, and blood and a pasty red-white material oozed out of the crack and onto the filthy concrete cellar floor. That ooze, I learned in medical school, was brain—Uncle Tom's brain was leaking out of his skull!

The doctor, who lived near, arrived from nowhere and started screaming, "I don't know what to do. I don't know." The doctor hunched his shoulders and looked at me and, shaking his head vigorously, said, "I don't know what to do. I really don't."

Then the doctor turned to Joan and asked for hydrogen peroxide. Joan nodded to me, and I got the brown bottle from the upstairs bathroom and handed it to the doctor, who poured it into the open skull and onto Uncle Tom's brain.

Suddenly, Uncle Tom shook all over, arching his back and pounding the cement with his head, bang-bang-bang, and in the process spreading the red-white ooze, his brain, all over the cement floor. Then Tom let out a gigantic gasp, stopped breathing, and lay there silent, and very still and very, very dead.

Yes, Tom O'Connor was dead. Dead for all time. Uncle Tom, who had survived trench warfare in World War I and gas attacks, died from a fall down a cellar stair. Life can be ironic. For good reason, Homer had the Olympian gods laughing at us humans. The weird thing was that Tom's death seemed utterly like a chance event. Does chance drown the worthy with the unworthy? The fit with the unfit? And why? I wondered. Was this the punishment for being mean to me during the fisticuffs lesson? His intention was good, and he did teach me an important lesson, which I learned at age six:

Never let your guard down.

That was not the only lesson I learned that Saturday. If I had to put the other lessons in a list, it would look like this:

1. Do no harm. The doctor was right and wrong. He was right when he said he didn't know what to do. He should have put his hands in his pockets and done nothing. Maybe Joan could have found someone who did know what to do. Maybe not. Maybe there was nothing to do. The doctor was

wrong to put peroxide on Uncle Tom's brain. Doing nothing would have been safer. In view of the peroxide-induced grand mal seizure, doing nothing would have been a lot safer. That's the truth.

2. Life is precarious and fragile. You can go from living to dead in the blinking of an eye or the slip of a foot on a cellar stair. If life could slip away so fast from the great and powerful Uncle Tom, war hero and boxing champ, what's going to happen to us mere humans? What's going to happen to me?

3. No matter how it happens, we all push up daisies. Death is inescapable, even if it is sometimes delayable. Tom probably could have delayed his death and lived longer, and not fallen if he had held on to the handrail. Since he fell backwards, it was obvious that he was ascending the stairs. He probably would not have fallen if he had been holding the handrail. In a certain sense, he failed to follow his own advice. He let his guard down. Some people think it is safer to go upstairs than down. So, some people hold on to the handrail going down but not up. Best to hold on both ways and avoid Uncle Tom's fate.

4. So far as I can make it out, our destiny is to perish, probably perish completely. I know there are other notions, very popular in certain quarters. Almost every religion offers some continued existence after death. And that offer probably helps keep those religions in business. From a scientific point of view, it is almost certain that when we die, we die forever. Uncle Tom probably can't see, hear, smell, taste, or even think anymore. He probably doesn't even know he's dead. We miss him, but he doesn't miss us.

We buried Uncle Tom, middleweight boxing champion of the British Army in Africa and war hero, in the family crypt in Calvary Cemetery. Sic transit gloria mundi. (Thus passes the glory of the world.) And yes, we buried Uncle Tom, as per his request, with his boxing gloves, just in case he might need them later on in the place where he has gone, where it's always double drill and no canteen. Uncle Tom might be sitting on the coals ready to give boxing lessons to poor damn souls. Me too. I may someday get another boxing lesson in Hell from Uncle Tom.

Next up is Doctor Andrew Mellissey, the family doctor who was our G.P. The idea of this encounter is to discuss what medicine was like in the past so we can compare and contrast it with what medicine is like now.

OUR FAMILY DOCTOR

ENCOUNTER EIGHT: OUR FAMILY DOCTOR

◆ ◆ ◆

Doctor Mellissey lived in a mansion in southeast Queens Village. His situation was like that of Doctor Lanza, but more elaborate. The west end of the mansion held the waiting room, the doctor's office with a real examining room, and a consultation room. There were office hours when you just dropped in to see the doctor, no appointment necessary or possible. Just like Doctor Lanza, there was no nurse, no receptionist, no forms to fill out, no insurance hassle. You arrived and waited until the doctor himself called you in.

Usually, Mom counted the number of people ahead of us and estimated the waiting time. She usually remarked, "Look at this—23 people here and each paying $8. The doctor is making a fortune."

Yes, unlike Doctor Lanza, Doctor Mellissey charged $8 for the visit and consultation. And unlike Doctor Lanza, Doctor Mellissey made house calls. Everybody paid the same except me. I paid nothing. After Doctor Mellissey found out I might be interested in becoming a doctor, I got (did you guess?) professional courtesy, and that meant no charge.

Mom didn't like it. "Please charge Mickey (Mickey = my nickname), it is only fair," she insisted. But the doctor shook his head no and smiled, "I can't charge him, professional courtesy. He might become a doctor."

And there never was a charge for my visits about my injuries on the track team—spiked in the Achilles tendon during the Queens championships, shin splints, multiple leg bruises (so many moms thought I might have leukemia), and so forth. I liked our family doctor. He was my friend and very interested in my going to medical school. But he wouldn't let me make house calls with him. "Too boring and unscientific. It might turn you off. My practice is not the real medicine. The real medicine is in the big centers like Columbia-Presbyterian, where they treat the really sick. If your I.Q. is higher than 125, you are wasting your life as a general practitioner."

Mom and Pop had different opinions about Doctor Mellissey.

Pop said, "For God's sake, Ol (Mom's name was Olga, but Pop called her Ol), why waste time and money on him. He knows practically nothing. The only thing he is good for is the name and address of the specialist."

"He's a doctor. Graduated from Downstate. He must know something, probably more than we do. I like him, and he takes good care of us, and he makes house calls. He got Mick through measles, mumps, chickenpox, German measles, whopping cough and he helped Jim (Jim = my brother) survive the skull fracture. So far, no polio. He knows his limits, too. He refused to set Mick's fractured arm and got the Health Insurance Plan surgeons to do it. And don't forget he saved Mick's life."

When Mom pulled that card (saved Mick's life), the argument ended.

She was talking about the time when I had measles and Doctor Mellissey made his usual house call. This was always a special event for us kids and for Mom. She cleaned the house the day before and made one of her special apple pies. No matter how sick, we kids were washed and dressed, propped up in bed, and told to look happy. In those days, there wasn't much medicine itself could do to help recovery. Survival depended more on nursing care than on the doctor's orders. And my mother was a devoted nurse whenever Jim or I or Pop got sick. She often neglected her own health, eating, and sleeping to keep watch over us. She was not frightened or deterred by the risk of catching the disease, and she never rested from delivering our three-square meals. No wonder at age 82 in intensive care at Houston Methodist I was wishing Mom was there with me sleeping in a cot in the room, helping my wife Ethel and my daughter Allegra take care of me and monitoring the doctor's orders, the nursing care, and the diet (Mom was big on food because she thought food was an important part of human nutrition). Wives and daughters are very important. Mothers are important too. Very important. No wonder on the beaches of Normandy, the wounded were calling for their mothers and the medics.

Back to the measles visit.

That day, I had a fever and the doctor suggested in addition to my usual treatment (a cup half tea and half Irish whiskey) that I might also benefit from an aspirin. I got the aspirin, and Mom and the doctor went downstairs for apple pie and coffee. Suddenly, I felt terrible, my face got swollen, and I had trouble breathing. I stumbled out of bed, tried to call for help, but no sound came from my throat. After that, I don't know what happened.

When I awoke, Doctor Mellissey was standing over me with a syringe in his hand.

He said, "Wow! That was close. No more aspirin for him. He's highly allergic. Lucky I was still here." Conclusion: If it hadn't been for the coffee and apple pie, the doctor would have left, and I would have died of a severe anaphylactic reaction to aspirin. Anaphylactic reaction is a severe, life-threatening allergic reaction that can happen in seconds or minutes after exposure to what you are allergic to. Common anaphylactic reactions occur in predisposed people to peanuts and bee stings. In my case, a single aspirin could kill me and almost did that day because I suddenly couldn't breathe and lost consciousness.

In that era, circa 1948, giving a child who has a viral illness aspirin for fever would have been O.K., maybe even the standard of care. Now aspirin for kids and teens is a no-no because of the possibility of Reye's syndrome. A syndrome is not a whore house at the airport. It's Greek—syn meaning together and drome meaning running. A syndrome is a running together of signs and symptoms. In Reye's syndrome, there is a sudden sickness that can cause major problems, including brain edema (edema = more fluid in tissue than there should be), liver failure, coma, seizures, and death. The root cause of the problem is not known. For some reason, the aspirin provokes a massive failure of the mitochondria, the cellular organelles that produce energy for every cell in the human body. Treatment is only supportive (and very expensive) because the root cause of the condition is not known and therefore can't be directly addressed. The best approach is not to produce the syndrome in the first place and the way to do that is by not giving aspirin.

That is why the current standard of care is directly the opposite of what it used to be. The reversal of thinking about health care and medical science is not unusual. Question: How come?

<u>Answer: Medicine is mainly unscientific because so little is actually really known.</u>

People, some people anyway, associate science with absolute truths that are immutable. Real scientists know that is not true.

<u>Science is a process for understanding nature and that process is continually uncovering new information, new truths. As the new information becomes available, the ideas of what was right and what was not so right must be adjusted to fit the new knowledge. That's progress, a form of self-correction.</u>

In 1948, Doctor Mellissey and, I am sure, no other person actually knew about Reye's syndrome until it was studied and exposed as a distinct danger of giving aspirin to children.

Let's face the facts. Biological and health sciences are soft sciences that are quite different from hard sciences like mathematics or physics or chemistry. With mathematics, two and two equals four. Ten years from now, two and two will equal four, and the same will be the case 100,000 years from now. When a drop of silver nitrate is added to a solution of sodium chloride a white precipitate of silver chloride will immediately appear. The same will happen 100,000 years from now. That is the triumphant exactness of chemistry. Physics is even more amazing with its mathematical laws that strangely and exactly predict natural phenomena.

Not so, this kind of consistency in medicine as the rather bleak history of medicine clearly shows. Things change. They have to change in any field where uncertainty is the rule. We just don't know enough about human physiology and biology to be sure about much of anything. Human biology and genetics are too messy and too complicated for our present state of understanding and knowledge.

All living things are physio-chemical machines. We just don't know enough about the chemistry and physics of living things to make completely accurate judgments about them using chemistry and physics, and mathematics.

Therefore, most of medicine involves guesswork and experiments. When I give a patient a medicine, I definitely have a strong reason to believe it will do good, but I know and I will be sure to tell the patient that we can't predict for sure what will happen. In a certain sense, all treatments are experiments. There is always the possibility of the improbable, the unexpected, or the unexpectable happening. The uncertainty bugs the public and, frankly, the uncertainty bugs me. But currently and well into the near future, that is the nature of nature and the state of the art of medicine.

Uncertainty bothered the public during the recent COVID-19 pandemic. Gradually, the public health authorities learned about transmissibility, severity, vulnerability of different people (the fat and the old), and the amount of protection expected from vaccination. Then the virus itself was continuing to evolve into different forms, some killed by antivirals or antibodies, and some not. A moving target is hard to hit. Some forms of the virus were affected by vaccination, some were not. The vaccines it turns out, in general, were not that great about preventing infection but they were effective in preventing serious illness and hospitalization, and death. Thus, the informed medical opinions had to evolve with the current data about what the virus was doing. Now we know that the original Messenger RNA vaccines were able to induce very good CD4+ and CD8+ T-cell responses, which made the vaccines effective in preventing severe disease and hospitalization, even when someone was infected with a new strain of the virus that had different spike proteins. But because the vaccines couldn't induce the production of neutralizing antibodies that matched the circulating strain's spike, vaccinated people could still get infected and pass the virus along to others. Medical advice had to change; the vaccine was good but not perfect. The vaccines often induced an unpleasant experience, causing flu-like side effects for a day or two in many people and more serious injuries in others. That was the nature of the state of the art. That was the unpleasant demand of the situation.

Further complicating the public's understanding was the issuing of stupid advice by President Trump and others who, believe it or not, suggested inhaling bleach would be a great treatment or that hydroxychloroquine would be effective. Trump had the personal touchiness of most propagandists; he believed that because he was sincere, therefore his opinions were always correct. Trump announced (and I actually saw a video of him announcing this) that he knew more than the doctors. He said this was especially remarkable because he had not gone to medical school. This is either an outright lie or the product of staggering ignorance. As a matter of fact, at the time, as a matter of hard scientific fact, extremely little was known by anyone about what to do about COVID-19.

Departures from reason and fact, and science and evidence by Trump did not help humanity deal with the reality of a pandemic and did cause great harm. The virus did not care what Trump said or believed. In Texas, it killed over 77,000 people. Worldwide, its first year killed over 3 million people. Nor did the virus care that Trump was president of the United States. The virus just continued to do its thing.

We now know bleach is not a good treatment for COVID, and it can cause great harm when inhaled. Extensive and expensive studies (most of which I believed were silly and unnecessary) proved that hydroxychloroquine does not work and caused some deaths. Wishful thinking and stupid ideas do not work when faced with a pandemic. And yet, it is amazing how those stupid ideas had so much traction, especially among the stupid. The other thing that bothers my sleep is that people believe Trump when they know he has been a liar his whole life long. Why people believe an inveterate liar like Trump is beyond the beyonds.

The sad news:

<u>If you think we are done with COVID, think again. COVID is not done with us.</u>

No way! This group of viruses has the unique ability to mutate at very rapid rates and thus escape treatments. SARS-COV-2 is so adept at changing the shape of its proteins that it did so just enough to evade the antibodies that the pharmaceutical companies designed to kill it. So, one by one, the FDA revoked antibody authorization because the antibodies no longer worked. Furthermore, for some reason, human immunity to this class of viruses does not last the way immunity lasts to other viruses like measles or smallpox. With the waning of immunity induced by vaccination or actual infection, we can expect a resurgence of COVID-19 sicknesses, maybe even another pandemic.

The World Health Organization estimates the vaccines saved the lives of 14 to 20 million people in their first year of use (ref: Lancet Infect. Dis. 2022,DOI: 10.1016/S1473=3099(22)00320-6). Much of the nuance on where the first COVID-19 vaccines succeeded and where they failed has been lost in the public discourse. It is easy to be critical today. But the vaccines did and will protect people. I believe the vaccines rescued society and probably saved the human race from extinction. People forget that if we didn't have those tools (vaccines, antivirals, antibodies), a lot more people would have died. Please don't forget the overloaded hospitals, the rationing of respirators, the shortage of nurses, and morgues so overfilled with corpses that refrigerated trucks were needed to store the dead.

I may be starting to sound like a broken record when I say that stupidity does not serve public health, but I guess stupidity is understandable when there is a pandemic and no effective therapy is on the scene.

Because of the desperate nature of HIV, people were willing to self-administer almost any substance or compound, including cucumber extract, anything really that gave a hint or rumor of being able to suppress the virus. Searching for an effective treatment, patients were willing to travel great distances and pay great prices for the hope of help. In July 1985, Rock Hudson went to France to get HPA-23, the experimental agent developed at the Pasteur Institute. HPA-23 proved ineffective, and Rock died of AIDS in 1985 at age 59.

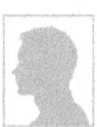

ENCOUNTER NINE

JIM AND I ALMOST DIE

ENCOUNTER NINE: JIM AND I ALMOST DIE

◆ ◆ ◆

Each summer we went somewhere. Whether it was Uncle Joe's (Mom's brother's) farm in Honesdale, Pennsylvania, or to the Miami Beach Eden Rock Hotel or across the planet. We toured Canada several times and even went to Labrador by car in the days when there were no gas stations, motels, or restaurants there. Pop would knock on some farmer's door and ask for gas, food, or lodging. One summer, we toured the United States for six weeks. Pop said the country was going to change a great deal, and he wanted us kids to see what it was like before the big change happened. That trip, in 1951, we had to carry our own water and, with the help of AAA (American Automobile Association), carefully plan where we would fuel, eat, and where we would sleep. We traveled the northern route west. I remember going through Kansas and not seeing a person, house, or animal the entire day. But I did see lots of corn and lots of roadside signs with bullet holes in them.

The trip was not boring. Painful, maybe, but not boring. Jim and I got San Joaquin Valley Fever in California and almost died on the way home. We stayed in the central valley for a while, trying to decide whether to go to Los Angeles or not. There was a polio epidemic in L.A., and Mom feared polio like she feared the devil. Many kids had come down with the paralytic form, and many were in iron lungs, and many had died. All of us kids knew someone who had contracted polio. People who speak against vaccination simply speak out of tremendous ignorance and prove they have not experienced a real polio epidemic. If you don't know what you are talking about, for heaven's sake, keep your mouth shut—zip it!

Mom prevailed, and we headed home as planned along the southern route, the famous Route 66. By the time we got to New Mexico, Mom and Pop lost their sangfroid and stopped at a hospital in Tucumcari, where both Jim and I were admitted. I was too sick to remember much of this, but I do remember the doctor standing at the bedside and telling us what was what. "Jim and Mick have Valley Fever that they caught by inhaling dust while you were at San Joaquin. This is an infection caused by a fungus (then a long word which was probably coccidiomycosis). There is no effective treatment. Antibiotics will not work. The kids will either die or recover. It won't make a difference if you leave or stay."

Mom: "What a relief. It's not polio then?"

Doctor: "Not polio. No polio, just a fungus in the lungs."

Mom: "Can we catch it?"

Doctor: "No. They can't transmit it. There has never been a reported case of transmission from one person to another. If the kids recover, they will be permanently immune and never again suffer the same infection. They may be left with lung scars, which will show up on X-rays and be read erroneously as *Old Inactive Tuberculosis*."

Since the doctor said it didn't matter if we stayed or left, we left.

Jim and I slept most of the way back to Queens Village, 15 to 18 hours a day. Yes, Jim and I suffered for two weeks in the back of the Chrysler. If we woke up, Mom would hand us a bottle of whiskey from the glove compartment, and we would take a swig and go back to sleep.

Review time: Was this encounter good medicine?

I say it was. The definite diagnosis removed fear of the unknown and was a major plus with Mom because the illness was not polio. There was no need to use antibiotics because the infection was not bacterial. That saved money and saved us from possible side effects. It also saved the general population from antibiotic resistance that might have developed from the senseless misuse of antibiotics. Further tests, X-rays, and so forth were not needed. No more tests! That too was a blessing.

Follow-up: The diagnosis and prognosis were correct. We recovered. On entering medical school, my skin test was still positive for coccidioidomycosis, the cause of Valley Fever, but my skin tests were negative for tuberculosis, histoplasmosis, and blastomycosis. My chest x-ray does show scars that have been read as old, inactive tuberculosis, but the skin test shows I never had T.B. Therefore, the scars on my lung are probably from valley fever.

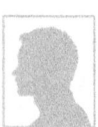

JIM SPENDS NEEDLESS TIME IN BED

ENCOUNTER TEN: JIM SPENDS NEEDLESS TIME IN BED

◆ ◆ ◆

Tragedy struck one day when Doctor Mellissey came to check Jim. Jim had a linear occipital skull fracture. He had been pulled down the steps of Hank Ulrich's home and hit the cement with the back of his head. Ernst, a neighborhood kid four years older than Jim and twice as big, was responsible. As Jim's big brother, I had a talk with Ernst, who admitted the assault. So, I beat Ernst up to teach him not to pick on little kids and not be a bully. It was shocking how easy it was to defeat Ernst, who had not been trained as a fighter. Uncle Tom would have been proud.

By the way, in that era (circa 1953), what was the treatment for Jim's linear skull fracture?

Answer: Bed rest for three months.

Yes, Jim had to stay in bed for three months and miss that amount of school. He did watch a lot of TV. Bed rest and observation for three months, and no other treatment. Also, Jim was not allowed to play the saxophone. I think the theory was that the pressure of blowing into the instrument might cause the brain to herniate through the skull fracture.

Nowadays, a linear skull fracture would be treated quite differently. Maybe there would be a few days of observation in the hospital to make sure there was no subdural hematoma (blood clot pressing on the brain) or infection and then the child would be back to normal activity in less than a week.

The past is a different country. They did things differently then. Three months in bed for a linear skull fracture was a wrong unnecessary treatment and these days would be considered highly questionable or even malpractice. But in the old days it was the standard of care.

Where was I before the truth broke in about Jim?

Oh yes, the tragedy that happened after Doctor Mellissey's visit to check Jim. I remember this exactly as if it were yesterday because of the profound impact it had on Mom and me. After the visit and the usual apple pie and coffee, we escorted Doctor Mellissey toward his car. Suddenly, by the front stoop, he turned, bowed his head, and with a sad face said, "I am leaving medicine. Too much paperwork. I bought a farm in New Jersey and will farm there. It is something I want to do, have to do. Sorry."

Ye gods! Even back then, too much paperwork.

Mom and I were speechless and helplessly watched Doctor Mellissey throw his black bag in the car, get in, and drive away. Mom was crying, and I think the doctor was either crying or close to it.

Conclusion: It was possible even in the old days for doctors to get burned out and leave the profession. The paperwork burden that Doctor Mellissey complained of was, I am sure, absolutely nothing compared to the paperwork burden doctors face today.

That was the last time we saw our family doctor, and the last time my family had a family doctor. Thereafter, we went to the Health Insurance doctors at Elmhurst Hospital in Elmhurst, Queens.

The Health Insurance Plan (HIP) was a kind of health insurance plan for New York City employees. My father, who thought New York ruled a quarter of the world, worked for the city as Chief Assistant District Attorney and was eligible to join the plan. Mom didn't like the plan because to get to see a doctor required a long trip to Elmhurst, and you had to make an appointment, and you first had to visit a local doctor HIP assigned, who did some paperwork and had to make a referral for you to get an appointment with the actual HIP doctor. Mom thought that the main idea of this kind of medical care was to collect the premiums and do nothing. Her opinion was confirmed when we consulted two surgeons about a four-inch scar I had on my left knee. I had run into a horseshoe stake at summer camp, and despite the camp doctor's advice that I should not swim with a fresh gaping wound, the next day was somewhat exigent. I had to swim in the camp swimming meet. To my troop I was a hero because I took first place in butterfly, but to the camp doctor I was a moron because I opened the wound so badly that it could no longer be safely sutured closed. The next encounter concerns the fate of the scar left by that wound.

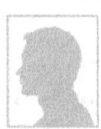

THE BEST TREATMENT IS NOTHING

ENCOUNTER ELEVEN: THE BEST
TREATMENT IS NOTHING

◆ ◆ ◆

After a few months, we got an appointment. Two H.I.P. surgeons explained that the scar might turn into a cancer sometime later, so that might be a reason to remove the scar, to prevent a cancer. "We can cut around the scar, remove it, and then suture the skin back. But that is a lot of work, and the whole thing might not heal." They advised, "Just live with the scar. When it turns into a cancer, come back and we'll take a look."

Whew! That was a relief. I liked the idea of no surgery, but I didn't like the idea of getting a sarcoma, the kind of cancer they predicted might occur. Mom was furious. "Thanks for nothing," she told them in a huff.

The scar is still there on my left knee, but so far, decades later, no cancer.

H.I.P. was an HMO before health maintenance organizations were popular. Mom was underwhelmed. "They're not interested in helping. Just like to collect the premiums and do nothing. What a racket!"

That is also my present opinion of H.M.O. They are not much interested in health, do not maintain it, but they are an organization, alright, an organization designed to extract money from the public. The less they do, the less they allow, the more they profit. Medicare Advantage programs are now under investigation for denying needed care or delaying care. There are all sorts of gimmicks used, among them preauthorization and preapproval. The doctors waste precious time on the phone trying to get an often-reluctant insurance company representative to preauthorize a test or prescription. And, get this, the preauthorization does not guarantee that they will pay! The companies consider preauthorization and actual payment as two different things. No kidding. Although my endoscopic operation (endoscope = a fiberoptic device used to look inside the gut) was preapproved and preauthorized, Blue Cross and Blue Shield of Texas refused to pay for it. So, I got stuck with a bill for $9,875.

The insurance company gimmick that I dislike the most is the step-up program. Step-up means that if you have a serious illness, you must try the cheaper (and often less effective) treatment before you can proceed to the more expensive, more effective treatment. Sometimes there are three step-ups you must try before you get to the most effective treatment. By that time, some people will die before they can step up and some may recover on their own or go to Norway or Mexico or France or the Czech Republic for care or operation or I.V.F., and some people will cough up the money themselves, if they can.

When I had klebsiella sepsis, the infectious disease doctor told me that, because my insurance wouldn't authorize payment, she would have to use oral and less effective antibiotics first and then, and only then, if the less expensive medicine didn't work, advance to the more effective more expensive intravenous antibiotic treatment. Naturally, I volunteered, and Ethel paid for the most expensive treatment, and we are happy we did so; otherwise, I might not be here to warn you about step-up programs. One of my good friends has been waiting over a year to step up to more effective treatment for his multiple myeloma. I hope he makes it.

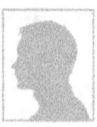

ANTONY DONN CHANGES MY LIFE

ENCOUNTER TWELVE: ANTONY DONN CHANGES MY LIFE

◆ ◆ ◆

At the end of the sophomore year at Columbia College, there was a week set aside for final examinations. These exams were important because they played a major role in determining your final grade in the courses you were taking. Like most of my fellow students, I was concerned about grades because if you didn't pass the course, you didn't get credit, and if you didn't get credit, you were one step further away from graduation.

But my worry about grades wasn't anywhere near my worry about going blind. Close your eyes and note what it is like not to see. One of my classmates had suddenly done just that—not closed his eyes—but actually had suddenly gone blind. Consequently, most of my fellow students and I were worried that the same might happen to us.

My fellow student had reported to the Columbia Health Care Service, which was at Saint Luke's Hospital across Amsterdam Avenue just east of our campus. He told the doctors he thought he was going blind. The doctors didn't think so. They thought he was worried about examinations. They were right, of course. He was worried about examinations as were we all. But the doctors were also wrong about his sight. He was going blind. He had acute glaucoma. Within a few days, he was completely and irreversibly blind for the rest of his life. Blind in both eyes.

That was a pity because glaucoma is treatable by lowering the intraocular pressure. If the treatment had been given on time, the blindness would not have happened. But now that it had happened, it was not reversible because permanent damage to the optic nerves had already occurred. The unrelieved pressure had permanently damaged the optic nerves. Medical science at that time and in our time has no way of fixing the damage and restoring sight. Stop and think about this. This is a tragedy of the first magnitude.

When the news got around, a lot of us started noticing difficulty with our eyes. I was no exception. Three days into the exam period, at about 9:15 in the evening, I was studying. There appeared a large, tangled brown spot in front of my right eye. The brown spot moved with the eye and seemed to get bigger and bigger the more I looked at it. The following morning, the physician at the Columbia Health

Service sent me right up to the Eye Institute at Columbia-Presbyterian Hospital for emergency consultation. They, at Saint Luke's, had missed the other student's glaucoma and weren't about to make the same mistake twice. Experience is a great teacher. Most physicians are one-step learners, especially if the mistake was a mistake of the magnitude that resulted in a permanently blind patient.

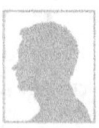

DOCTOR DONN KNOWS THE ENLIGHTENMENT IS MAN'S EMERGENCE FROM SELF-IMPOSED NONAGE

ENCOUNTER THIRTEEN: DOCTOR DONN KNOWS THE ENLIGHTENMENT IS MAN'S EMERGENCE FROM SELF-IMPOSED NONAGE

◆ ◆ ◆

The doctor I saw was Anthony Donn. His first question was, "What are you reading?"

"Emanuel Kant's essay, *What is the Enlightenment.*"

This was my preparation for the final examination in a course that I was taking, a four-credit course, pompously and verbosely entitled *Contemporary Civilization in the West: Readings in and Discussion of Western Literature and Philosophy.*

At that point, Doctor Donn told me that the enlightenment was man's emergence from self-imposed nonage and that nonage was a willful obedience to the will of another. He knew that the Western world owed much of its values and mores to the *Enlightenment's* faith in human reason and its assertion of individual rights.

Holy cow! Donn summarized in a nutshell exactly what the essay was about and what Kant thought the Enlightenment was about. So here we had a physician, an ophthalmologist, who was probably a long way out of college and yet able to quote exactly what Kant had said in his famous essay. Very impressive.

Even more impressive was Dr. Donn's examination of my eye. After he had finished, he drew exactly what I was seeing. "This is a persistent hyaloid artery that you have had since birth. You will carry it to your death. The hyaloid artery in embryonic life runs right through the center of the eye. In most cases, it is resorbed so that it can't interfere with vision. It will have no more adverse effect on your sight than it is having now."

"But how come I am seeing it now when it has been in my eye all the time?"

"You have probably been seeing it on and off and not paying it mind. You knew what happened to your classmate, so you paid more attention. The brain usually ignored it as it often does until you began to fear you were going blind. You are not going blind. Everything is going to be O.K. You can ignore it. Or you can see it as you wish."

Wow! That was a relief.

On the way back to Columbia, while on the A-train, I had what some people might call an epiphany. I didn't have anything wrong with my vision and yet I felt enormously better. Doctor Donn had made me feel enormously better just by talking to me and telling me what was what. He didn't even give me a medicine or a treatment. He just gave assurance. But the assurance was real power. It was the power of medicine to help me feel better. Amazing!

I thought about the possibility that if I had had something wrong of what great things medicine might do for me to fix me. Donn was right, too. I could see the persistent artery, and I could make it disappear as I saw fit. There was no question about it: Medicine was a powerful force. Doctor Donn did mention that if the acute glaucoma had been diagnosed in time, it could have been easily treated and vision saved. The blindness could have been completely prevented. Imagine that power! The power to save a person's vision. Tears rushed to my eyes thinking about it. They still do. Big tears.

When I got off the A-train at 116 Street and Broadway, I walked across the campus and decided as I passed a statue of Alma Mater (that great big copper statue of a woman, the Kindly Mother, Our Kindly Mother, presiding over the Columbia campus), that by God I was going to be a doctor! I was going to have that power, the power of medicine, the power to heal, the power to reassure.

Straight to Hamiliton Hall, I marched, climbed four flights of stairs, and blew into my advisor's office. My advisor was the very famous American historian James P. Shenton! My father loved Professor Shenton and was sure not to miss a single lecture on American history that Shenton put on TV each week. And me, woe is me. I was about to make the great professor sick!

Shenton seemed to sense the danger, for he looked at me with a frightened face, stood up behind his desk, and asked in an excited voice, "Patten, for God's sake, what's wrong?"

My head bowed in disgrace. In those days, admitting you wanted to be a doctor, admitting you wanted to be pre-med, wanting to cure people and relieve suffering was déclassé. Part of me, too, felt that way, a little ashamed of what I had decided.

Believe it or not, I said, "Professor Shenton, I have degenerated into a pre-med." Exactly that. *Degenerated.*

About this sudden transformation, Shenton was not happy. He knew my father was the Chief of Homicide Prosecutions in Queens and a politician. He knew my Uncle, Senator Patten, was also a politician. Shenton knew my family expected me to be a politician. Shenton knew, as did we all know, that in that era the way to enter politics was through the law. Shenton also had the usual Columbia College bias against pre-med students because they were derisible grubs, grubs for grades.

Although medicine is an honorable profession, Shenton and my father and my Uncle, Senator Patten, all felt that doctors were like shoe repair people; sometimes necessary, but in a basically boring job. Doctors made a decent living, even in depressions. But the real thing, the real deal, the thing that changes the course of history, that affects the health and welfare of millions, is not medicine. The real thing is (did you guess?)—the real deal is politics.

And so it was with considerable disdain that my advisor, Professor James P. Shenton, my father and my Uncle Senator Patten looked down on the medical profession in general and on my transformation, in particular.

Pop said, "You have disgraced yourself, but I won't cut you off. Everyone has the right to do what they want with their life. If you want to waste your life taking care of the weak, the sick, the tired, the hurt, the wounded, the drunks, the drug addicts, the kooks, and the poor at all hours of the day and night, that's your problem."

I am not exaggerating their views. To them, medicine was a waste of talent. With less disdain, they would have looked down on me if I had asked for a sex change. In their view, my transition from pre-law to pre-med was worse than a transition from being a man to being a woman. No kidding!

Shenton wasn't going to give up. He had an idea. "This might be a sudden psychosis or some other mental aberration brought on by the stress of examinations."

He got on the phone and called for an emergency consultation at Columbia-Presbyterian Medical Center, this time at the Psychiatric Institute with a psychiatrist.

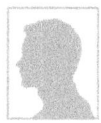

PSYCHIATRIC WISDOM

ENCOUNTER FOURTEEN: PSYCHIATRIC WISDOM

◆ ◆ ◆

At the Psychiatric Institute, Doctor Donald Kornfield listened for eight minutes to the Donn story, the train story, and to the Shenton scene. He shook his head and called Shenton. "The kid wants to be a doctor. What the hell is wrong with that?"

That is how it came to pass that I degenerated into a pre-med student, and I was happy for it. My major changed from American History to Chemistry. That made my life easier. There was far less reading in chemistry, and my laboratory experience at home from age 10 helped. In chemistry, I could just coast because it was easier to understand and made more sense than history. Chemistry was more my kind of discipline. It was actually scientific, with absolutely predictable reactions, all of which were more interesting to me and much more fun than reading the bland history of the whiskey rebellion. I especially enjoyed the beautiful colors of qualitative analysis, like the blue of cobalt or the green of copper salts, and with chemistry, there were the advantages of making explosives. I loved making explosives, and I loved blowing things up.

I graduated with 56 credits in chemistry, all A or A+ work. They elected me to the National Chemical Honor Society and to the American Chemical Society. In 1961, I was one of twelve members of the junior class elected to Phi Beta Kappa. That was the top two percent of our class. My best friend, Walter Hilse, was first in the class. I was second, and my former roommate, Peter Winn, was third.

Before closing this chapter, I want to mention that at no time did I wait to see either Doctor Donn or Doctor Kornfeld or the doctor at the Columbia Health Service. No forms were filled out. There was no nurse or secretary to greet me. No physician assistants. There was no discussion of payment. In fact, it never entered my mind that payment might be involved. And there was no insurance involved. No many-paged release forms were signed or even existed. No official medical record was made of the encounters. None! All this makes me think that today at least some of the efficiency of treating patients might be compromised by all the rigmarole, red-tape, and forms as well as by the time involved in making a medical record. All that added time and effort might be part of the cause of the current high cost of medical care. What do you think?

Coda to the Doctor Donn story:

At one of the College of Physicians and Surgeons reunions, I gave the keynote address on the new information and new treatments for myasthenia gravis. The master of ceremonies who introduced me was Doctor Antony Donn himself. He didn't remember me, but I remembered him, and I told the assembled group the Donn story and how Donn was responsible for my going into medicine. Doctor Donn was visibly and emotionally touched by, as he said, "by your story and subsequent achievement," and since that time, we have been good friends. He has written letters about how he considers my conversion from law to medicine one of the highlights of his life. His very poor handwriting in these letters shows that he also had, like me, a progressive education. And yes, Tony and I have talked on the phone about his personal problems, which shall remain secret. He invited me and my family to his retirement home in Vermont, the Burklyn Mansion on Darling Hill Road, East Burke. We have not yet visited him and his wife Linda, but we hope to help him celebrate his 100th birthday in 2026. We will help him celebrate, if and only if, he has not by that time crossed the river Styx.

Burklyn Mansion has an interesting history, which goes back to Darling, the big businessman who built the mansion and purchased and developed over 1400 surrounding acres in this little Vermont town, population 132. If you wish, take a look at what the mansion is like on YouTube. Donn's is a palace, and palaces, whether they are little ones, as Donn's, with its 35 rooms, or Buckingham or vast Fontainebleau, are all alike; choked with pride, and according to Doctor Donn (private communication), altogether tedious. He regrets buying the place, but I am sure will take pride in showing its enduring charms to Ethel and me.

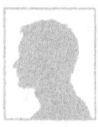

ENCOUNTER FIFTEEN

CLASSIC MEDICINE IN A BYGONE ERA

ENCOUNTER FIFTEEN: CLASSIC MEDICINE IN A BYGONE ERA

◆ ◆ ◆

The first thing I noticed was that the green and white highway signs looked amazingly beautiful. The green seemed brighter and greener than I had ever seen before, and on highway 45 (Gulf Freeway), the green stood out from the signs and seemed to dance, scintillate, and shimmer in the air. Although I was driving to work, I pulled over, actually stopped to admire the extreme beauty of these green road signs. Transfixed and mesmerized by the beauty of green highway signs—that's what I was. But why?

Staring at the green signs did have an interesting aftereffect. The world now looked rose colored, a vie en rose. This after image is caused by the fatigue of the overused green receptors that need some rest while the red retinal receptors sleep. The reverse effect is seen by heart surgeons. They stare at bright red blood for hours, and when they leave the operating room, the usually white hospital walls appear—you guessed it—green. Known as "afterimage," the alien green comes from the physiology of the retina, seemingly out of nowhere, to counterbalance the depleted red cones disproportionately stimulated. The green cones, having napped during surgery, are now on the scene. All this is a natural phenomenon freely available to anyone who wishes to study it. As for me, I prefer looking at the pinkish-peach sky to looking at headache-inducing puke greenish thrum. How about you?

Next, I noticed no matter how high I turned up the air conditioner in my Lincoln, I still felt hot. Bayway Lincoln checked things out and said nothing was wrong, so I bought a new Lincoln, hoping its air conditioner would work better.

Nope. The problem remained and, in fact, got gradually worse. Even with the A/C on MAX, I was hot and often sweating.

My usual appetite got bigger, much bigger. At home for dinner, I ate two steaks and cleaned up anything left over on the kids' and Ethel's plates. Despite the large intake of food, my weight declined from 158 to 140 pounds. I didn't like what I saw in the mirror. I was beginning to look like a malnourished Asian. My muscles were getting smaller. I was looking like a weakling and the reason I looked that way was that I was a weakling.

About that time, I noticed difficulty getting off the toilet, indicating the proximal muscles of my lower extremities were weak, and my grip strength, which I checked every night, was in steep decline, going from 183 pounds to 86. There were multiple muscle twitches and increased reflexes, so I diagnosed myself as having amyotrophic lateral sclerosis (ALS), a fatal nervous system disease. As there was (and still is) no real treatment for this disease, I decided just to let myself drift out. This was a mistake. A physician who diagnoses himself has a fool for a patient and a fool for a doctor.

Strangely, the routine paperwork in my medical practice got done much faster, and I published several new research papers in a jiffy. Never had I been so efficient and productive in such a small amount of time. My mood was great, naturally high. But why? What the heck was going on?

Saturdays found me refereeing at the kids' soccer game. Within ten minutes of blowing the whistle, I was short of breath, shorter of breath than any player. I had to drop out of that job because I just couldn't keep up with the kids.

Baylor College of Medicine used to have a lunchroom for faculty. The camaraderie and the conversations were important, but we never discussed our problem cases. This was a nice place to relax in the middle of a busy day, and the food was excellent. Usually, I ate with Fran, the Baylor veterinarian, and Peter Kohler, the chief of the Endocrine Division of the Department of Medicine. It was a pleasant lunch, even though Fran smoked at the end of her meal. Smoking at lunch in a medical school is now a no-no, but at the time, it seemed perfectly normal and acceptable, especially since Fran looked very happy and very sexy when she smoked her Benson and Hedges cigarette.

One day, Pete looked at my double lunch plate (twice what anyone else was eating) and my four desserts and said, "Bernie, you're hyperthyroid." I replied, "No, Pete, I'm just hungry."

Pete: "I will prove it. After lunch, come to my lab and I will examine you and draw blood."

Pete did a history and physical exam and pointed out several physical findings in hyperthyroidism (thyroid gland making too much thyroid hormone), including plumber's nails (nails with blank spaces under the nails) and a rapid small-amplitude tremor of my outstretched hands, which he said was characteristic of hyperthyroidism. I told him the same thing I told my secretary and the operating room nurses who had pointed out the same tremor, "Looks like I need a vacation."

Pete did a history and physical exam, but never wrote anything down, and of course, there was no charge. The technician drew the blood tests, and there was no charge for the tests. In fact, charges were never even thought about. It would have never occurred to me that Pete might charge me or that the tests would cost something. We, in that era, did not think in that mode.

That evening, I told Ethel that the chief of Baylor Endocrinology said I was hyperthyroid, and she said, "hyperthyroid—no, hyper sexed—yes—you are definitely hyper sexed."

Pete was right. I was severely hyperthyroid, and that was the diagnosis, not ALS. Everything was now explainable: the weight loss, the muscle weakness, the shortness of breath, the tremor, the feeling hot, the beautiful green colors and the remarkable speed of production in routine paperwork, the natural high, the very productive medical research, and so forth. The question now was what to do, if anything.

Pete said he would take care of me. He started a beta blocker called guanidine, a medicine no longer available. I did feel less hot, and the tremor was less. But I was still hyper. He then gave me methimazole, which did seem to tone down the hyper, but not enough. So, Pete switched to propylthiouracil (PTU), a drug that tends to prevent the production of thyroid hormones. This worked very well for three months, and I was pretty much on the road to normal when I developed total body hives and had to stop the PTU. I was allergic to PTU, the only hyperthyroid medicine left.

Ugh! Now what?

Pete presented my case at Methodist Hospital's Internal Medicine grand rounds, attended by over 100 internists. I answered questions and explained how much I enjoyed being hyperthyroid, especially the increased vividness of colors and the lack of fatigue. I liked the feeling of being wired (hyperactive) all the time, and I like the hypersexuality that was part of this so-called disease.

The internists were not impressed. They were extremely critical of Pete's management, and I was shocked by the vitriol and viciousness. I was lucky I was in a good mood; otherwise, I would have punched some of the more severe critics. No one should say such things about Pete Kohler, my doctor.

As a group, the internists claimed the severe hyperthyroidism should have been treated much more aggressively and that Pete had endangered my life because a delay in treatment could have produced a fatal heart arrhythmia.

And this was the most unkindest cut of all: All of them voted that I should have my thyroid gland ablated by radioactive iodine 131 (RAI-131) that day or the next day.

After grand rounds, Pete and I had a pow-wow.

Pete: "Holy cow. I apologize. I thought you had a small thyroid gland, and there was a reasonable chance you might go into remission. I was shocked that all voted for radioiodine and blamed me for endangering your life by not treating you with it. Mea culpa, mea culpa, mea maxima culpa." Pete had been an altar boy.

Me: "Pete, you are my doctor. Tell me what to do and I will salute." And at this point, I actually did salute him. "I don't like the idea of radiation because I know there is no safe dose, and probably in the future, I will get cancer caused by the treatment. I already got too much radiation at Brookhaven National Laboratory when I worked for the Atomic Energy Commission. Also, after RAI-131, I will be hypothyroid for life and will need thyroid pills every goddam day. Besides, the group didn't understand the benefits of hyperthyroidism. I don't mind feeling wired. In fact, I like it. I like the vivid colors, especially green and blue, and I like sex twice a day (sometimes actually three times a day) and very big meals."

Dear reader, notice how being a doctor does influence how you accept or don't accept a treatment. Doctors are fully aware that things can and often do go wrong. Every intervention has a chance of causing side effects. Don't believe me? Read the package insert that comes with your next prescription. In England, the side effects are call consequents. They are consequent because they naturally follow from the treatment.

Pete said nothing. Instead, he grabbed my neck and felt my thyroid gland. Then he shook his head. "Definitely small gland. I still think you may go into remission. In fact, I would bet on it. Let's just do nothing. You can't take any of the thyroid meds so that's that. You are tolerating the disease and you even like some of the effects. Over the long term, though, the hyper will rot your bones and damage your heart. If there is any stress in your life, try to eliminate it. Cutting stress might help induce remission."

Ummm! Stress! You bet. There was stress alright. Lots of stress.

Doctor DeBakey fired Doctor John Sterling Meyer, the chair of the neurology department and I, as vice-chair, was running the department, a job I hated. The other faculty members were such crybabies always asking for things. One complained his parking spot wasn't as close to the school as another faculty member. Another wanted money for another technician because he found out another faculty member had one technician more than he had. One faculty member was doing vaginal exams on all new women patients regardless of their age so we needed a committee to evaluate that practice in view of the complaints from some women. And then there were those boring faculty meetings where most of the other doctors loved to hear themselves (most of them are fools) talk while I felt I was bleeding to death. Committee meetings! I can't take them anymore. I am too much absorbed in my research and in patient care to waste time on morons.

Help! I asked for relief. Administration is not my thing.

Doctor DeBakey assigned Robert Williams, the chair of Psychiatry, as acting chair of neurology, and that cut my stress and administrative work way down. I loved seeing patients and doing research, but administration was not my thing. I didn't like telling people what to do, and I didn't like saying no to requests, even the reasonable ones. The department resources were extremely limited in part because Doctor DeBakey had a scotoma about neurology. Doctor DeBakey famously summarized his opinion of neurology: "If you can't cut on it or cut it out, what good is it?"

Two weeks later, after Doctor Williams took over, Pete checked my blood. It was normal, and I was taking no medicines! Was I in remission? A spontaneous remission? Recheck a month later, same result, all normal. Three months later, same result. Clinically, I was back to my old self, gaining weight and strength and seeing colors normally.

Pete decided to check thyroid hormone levels every six months. We did that for eight years. All my subsequent blood thyroid hormones have been smack in the middle of the normal range. This was a true remission, and Pete saved me the trouble of getting RAI-131 and saved me the trouble of taking thyroid pills for the rest of my life. Thank you, Peter Kohler. You gave me the advantage of no treatment (and thus gave me a chance for spontaneous remission), and you gave me the advantage of not having to take thyroid pills for the rest of my life. That was 50+ years ago. One pill a day times 50 years is 18,250 pills. Fifty years is 600 months. The current cost of a month's supply of levothyroxine, according to Amazon.com, without insurance, is $49.50. So, 600 times $49.50 comes to $29,700, enough money to pay for a nice vacation in the South Pacific.

What's the big deal?

How crowded is your pillbox? Take a look. With age often comes an increase in the number of medicines and in the number of pills you take. According to Joanne Doyle Petrongolo, a pharmacist at Harvard-Affiliated Massachusetts General Hospital, about one-third of patients aged 62 to 85 take five medications per person per day. In the higher risk, that is the sicker population, the number rises to 15 meds or more per person. Besides the hassle and inconvenience, taking multiple pills drives up costs to you and your insurance company. And remember this: The more medications you take, the greater the chance of side effects. And the greater the chance of errors taking the medications (especially errors of omission), and the greater the chance of drug interactions and quality of life issues. Talk with your doctor. Tell him/her you feel like you're taking too many pills. Ask if they can be reduced. But never downsize on your own or stop a medicine abruptly. Stopping some meds suddenly can have grave effects and can even cause death. My Uncle Fred decided he didn't need insulin for his Type I diabetes. So, he stopped the insulin. Two weeks later, Uncle Fred was no longer with us.

Follow-up on RAI-131.

Studies have documented that people who had no evidence of cancer when they got RAI-131 developed more cancers than expected, mainly breast cancers and colon cancers, which are no fun. Repeat studies showed again a small but definite increase in cancer in the RAI-131-treated group compared to a matched control group not treated. I know any radiation is unsafe, and I worry about the health consequences of all the chest x-rays and CT scans that are being done these days. CT (computed tomography) especially hits you with a big dose of radiation.

Doctor Peter Kohler was elected to the National Academy of Sciences in 1996, a great honor which he deserves. But the nay-sayers have not gone away. Despite the excellent result from doing nothing, Pete's management was severely critiqued at a recent meeting of the retired physicians' association. A member of Pete's own department, now retired, shook his head and said, "You should have gotten the RAI, the standard of care. Your remission was probably due to antithyroid antibodies."

What's the lesson?

I don't know. Perhaps following the protocol treatment for each and every patient is not such a good idea. Cookbook medicine is not appropriate for everyone under every situation. Treatments should be tailored to the individual patients, their individual needs, and interests. These days, I regret to report, the doctor whose job in the golden age demanded critical thinking, integrity, and guts is much less in evidence, because modern doctors are closely bound to the computer and subject to elaborate systems that direct their work. The systems dictate process and results, and doctors are evaluated on their adherence to the system. Independently minded doctors are repeatedly and severely criticized for using discretion and judgment in evaluating and treating individual patients. That's wrong! You agree or not?

Perhaps, Peter Kohler was smarter than any of the internists and had a better understanding of my personal needs than the group of internists at medicine grand rounds did. That's true because Pete more or less predicted the remission. Also, I liked and took to heart his advice about stress. Whether stress reduction played a role in the remission is debatable, but it certainly improved my life and outlook and happiness. I learned administration was not my thing, and I resolved to avoid it as much as possible.

Although RAI-131 is still a major treatment for hyperthyroidism, along with surgery and pills, there are now serious discussions about the cancer problem, and patients must be made aware of the risks involved.

In my view, another major lesson is that very effective medicine was practiced without any written record. That proves to me that medical record keeping is not necessary for a good result. I wonder if all this modern attention to record-making and record-keeping might be a waste of precious time and energy. Some of it I know diverts attention away from the actual patient, and I feel probably also diverts attention away from effective solving of medical problems, especially the more complex and difficult problems. Some of what you just read has to be true. And some of it has to be driving up costs, and some of it is contributing to physician burnout. Records are important in medical research, but I have an idea that for the bulk of routine medical care, they are a waste of time and energy.

Could it be that the records are really mainly for the benefit of the insurance companies? Could it be that the written record has much more to do with billing than with actual medical care and medical effectiveness? What really is the benefit for so many doctors to be spending nights and weekends on their charts when they could be better off reading the medical journals or having fun, or sleeping? I will discuss in part two what is wrong with modern medical billings, which proves to be that almost anything that can go wrong might actually go wrong.

Coda: Case in point

As chief of the nerve and muscle division at Baylor College of Medicine, I took care of other faculty members. For example, the chair of another department noticed he couldn't chop as much wood at his country home, and he was having trouble getting off the toilet and climbing stairs. I examined him in his office and we did tests. The blood testosterone was zero, which was the weakness's probable cause. Treatment with the male hormone solved the problem and restored the doctor to normal. Never was any written record made of this encounter, nor was there ever any discussion of payment for anything. There was never any form or insurance check, and no nurse or other person separated me from the patient. That was just the way some medicine was practiced in the bygone era, which some physicians (myself included) call the golden age of medicine. What was normal for that time and those circumstances worked, and often worked well.

My tap sisters (the ladies I tap dance with) think they get much more humanistic attention and better results from nurse practitioners than from the routine visits to a doctor. In their view, modern doctors need to learn how to relate directly to patients on the patient's level, the way nurse practitioners do. "The nurses listen better and charge less; order fewer tests and are more interested in solving problems than in consulting the computer. For major problems, we need big doctors and hospitals, but for the small stuff, nurses are better."

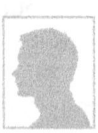

NETWORKING PAYS

ENCOUNTER SIXTEEN: NETWORKING PAYS

◆ ◆ ◆

In the middle of my last year of residency, the draft board in Jamaica, Queens, sent a letter telling me that I would be drafted into the United States Army in July of 1970 and would be assigned to the infantry in Vietnam, except under the condition that I volunteered for a commission. The draft board said that in the case that I qualified for a commission, they would let me satisfy my two-year draft obligation as an officer and physician. I had a wife and two children, and I was being drafted at age 29. The draft board assured me that physicians were draftable until age 36.

So, I volunteered for service during the Vietnam War and went into the Army Reserves as a lieutenant. The army would let me finish residency in neurology and the fellowship in human memory.

Canada was too cold for me. And who would have predicted that President Carter would pardon the draft dodgers? Thus, the record shows I volunteered for service during the Vietnam War when, actually, I did, but under duress.

My problem now was to find a job for the academic year from July 1, 1969, to July 1, 1970.

A neurosurgeon in Queens was willing to pay me a nice salary of $15,000 a year (my salary as a resident that year was $4,500), but he had some fixed ideas about the management of neck and back cases that did not coincide with my own. Neurosurgeons tend to operate, and I preferred to just treat the patients with rest, pain pills, muscle relaxants, heating pads, massage, and tincture of time. Overwhelmingly, the patients treated this way recovered nicely in about six weeks. It didn't seem to matter whether they rested or went about their usual activities. The healing forces of nature, in most cases, worked as well as surgery. So that job in Queens was out. I couldn't be a coolie and kowtow to a surgeon if I didn't believe that most of the patients needed his ministrations.

As everyone knows, children can be an unnatural burden on their parents. For that reason, parents have invented a type of jail called "school" to keep the kids under control. But what do you do on weekends when school is out?

Ethel and I had a solution.

I would watch the kids on Saturday and she would watch them on Sunday. Saturdays, she could go where she wished and do what she wanted. To this day, I don't know what she did or where she went. But I know what I did on Sundays.

I went to the reading room of the New York Academy of Medicine and read the medical journals. This might sound strange to you, but that is what I did. A busman's holiday, but for me it was a true pleasure. I love reading scientific journals. I love learning about the new things coming out. We are living in amazing times. Science is advancing at an amazingly rapid pace.

Ethel knows my true ambition is to be a cultured scholar, and I have often told her I would be content just to read all day and all night. Usually she says, "After a few hours you will get hungry and want food, and sometimes you will need to answer the call of nature by emptying your bladder, and sometimes you will want to sleep and sometimes you will want to screw." Actually, she didn't say screw; she used the F-word, which means the same.

She did have a point there, especially about eating. Ethel knows I would never kill for money or sex, but I would kill for food.

Even as a medical student, I used to steal away from the wards and read in the stacks of the medical library of the College of Physicians and Surgeons. There, usually on a Wednesday afternoon, I would huddle among the medical journals. I would randomly pull a journal off the shelf and read. As early as 1930, there were articles about smoking causing cancer of the mouth and lungs. Imagine that! President Grant's physician gave it for his opinion that Grant's mouth cancer was caused by "smoking too many cigars." There were lots of lessons in the old literature. That was one of them.

Some of the old investigators did outlandish things. One article took a cat and sewed up its anus. The cat got very unhappy and very sick. After that, the investigator measured an increase in blood ammonia that got bigger and bigger until the cat died. Conclusion: Suture of the anus caused ammonia to build up in the blood and the ammonia was probably toxic. I know this seems obvious to us, now, that suturing the anus closed was going to produce problems for the cat or for that matter for any animal. But evidently it took research to figure that out.

Original publications by famous doctors were sometimes laughable. Most of Freud would not be accepted today, especially his interpretation of dreams, as his work, according to modern standards, is not scientific. In fact, most of Freud is downright stupid. The past is a different country. They did things differently there. Here's another example: John Hughlings Jackson published a paper on *Singing by Speechless Children* (1866) in which he did not personally observe any singing in either of the two children he reported. Yet, Jackson is considered the founder of British neurology.

It was in the vaults of medical libraries that I gained a sense of history, which I am trying to pass on to you, a feeling for the flimsy nature of medical articles and medicine in general, and a sense of the ridiculous. One hundred years from now, the medicine of our era will look just as absurd and shameful, especially chemotherapy, which will (I hope) go the way of electroconvulsive shock (on the rise again, I recently read, which is disturbing, sorry), insulin shock, and frontal lobotomy. The literature of medicine proves that medicine is mostly guesswork. No! I retract that statement. The literature of medicine proves that all medicine involves guesswork… more or less.

One Sunday afternoon, at about 3 o'clock in the reading room of the New York Academy of Medicine, my bladder was full, and I needed to go to the men's room to pee. Pee is a medical term for micturition.

In those days, the reading room was on floor three and the men's room was on floor two. To get from floor three to floor two, you did not walk down a flight of stairs. Oh, no. You took the elevator. The elevator was not self-service. It was run by a special person called the elevator man. So being part of the era, I stepped into the elevator and asked for floor two. The elevator man did not move. Instead, he shook his head and pointed in the direction of the hallway indicating we were to wait for an old codger who was approaching. This codger was well dressed, and looked wealthy and healthy. He was much taller than I and in his eighties. Using one stick (the old medical term for a cane), he moved somewhat slower than usual but with dignity. He was headed to the same floor as I was and, in fact, was headed to the same place as I was—the men's room. In fact, he was headed to the men's room to do the same thing I was to do—namely, pee.

In the elevator and on the way, the old guy was ranting and raving, saying things in language typical for New York, but which might offend non-New Yorkers. I will paraphrase and shorten his discourse:

"I've been in this fucking reading room for three hours trying to find something that will help the failing memory of my friend. Medical science hasn't a goddamn thing to offer."

I said nothing. Just looked up at him while both of us peed in adjacent urinals.

"I have a good mind to pay some young physician to take a year off and study human memory to see if anything might be done to help."

I turned and looked up at him. As mentioned, he was much taller than I, and I had to strain my neck to look at him squarely in the face. He looked sincere. "How much money are we talking about?"

A beat as he paused and stared down his nose at me. He smiled and seemed interested.

After a pause, he asked, "Would $20,000 do it?"

When we had finished, we washed our hands and shook on the deal. I would take a year to study memory, and he would pay me $20,000 for my trouble. His name was Milton Raisbeck. He was a retired New York City cardiologist. No papers were signed, but I had no doubt that he would do what he said he would do, and I am sure he had no doubt that I would hold up my end of the bargain. That's the way things were done in that era, doctor to doctor. Doctor Raisbeck trusted me, and I trusted him, implicitly and explicitly.

The next day, Doctor Raisbeck called. "There's a snag. My accountant says it would be better if I donated the money to the New York Academy of Medicine. That way, I get a tax deduction. The Academy, in turn, would give the money to you as a fellowship, and that way, six grand of it would be tax-free to you."

"Whatever you say, Doctor Raisbeck."

The next day, Doctor Raisbeck called again. "There is another snag. The academy says they would have to advertise the fellowship throughout the city and they would have to accept applications from other physicians.

But, of course, the fellowship goes to you."

"Whatever you say, Doctor Raisbeck."

"Good. Here's what I want you to do. I want you to send a letter to the New York Academy of Medicine. In the letter, you are to say, 'If I am selected as the fellow, I will spend one year studying human memory.' That is to be your entire research plan and your entire fellowship application. Got it? Sign it, Bernard M. Patten, MD. Don't add that you are the chief resident neurologist at the Neurological

Institute of the Columbia-Presbyterian Medical Center. I will take care of the rest. Okay?"

"Whatever you say, Doctor Raisbeck."

Oh yes, Doctor Raisbeck somehow found out I was the chief resident neurologist. That doesn't sound like much, but it is a lot. This was the only time in my life that I had real power. I controlled the schedule for all the fellows and residents, arranged the conferences, and taught the third-year medical students. I even fired two residents, Priest because he had moon burn (too much moonlighting), and Roses for failing to take care of a patient in status epilepticus. I had my own office, which was lined by pictures of all the previous chiefs, most of whom were already famous neurologists and some of whom were already dead. I had my own secretary who had a separate office. Her name was Mary Anne.

It took Mary Anne three minutes to prepare, type up, and mail my fellowship application. They tell me that applications these days are wordier. That is too bad. Research is reaching out into the unknown. If you already know what you are going to do and you put that in writing in your application, the scope of your exploration of the unknown will be limited. You might, by that method, make some limited progress, but real breakthroughs are unlikely.

After she took care of my letter, Mary Anne, who usually wore a size zero mini miniskirt, told me she wanted to marry a doctor. She wanted to marry the richest resident Columbia had. "Who might that be?"

I told her about Warren, one of my first-year residents, whose family I think owned a chain of restaurants in Canada. "Ask him to come see me. I want to date him."

Subsequently, they married and have lived happily. Warren went on to become Chair of Neurology at Mount Sinai Medical School.

The only other time I played matchmaker was when Danny Sciarra's wife died. Danny came to me and said, "I need a wife. Do you know anyone around here suitable?"

"There's a nice radiology technician in the basement. She's Italian too, a little overweight, so she is probably a good cook."

Danny went down and talked to her. Soon thereafter, they were married.

There is another marriage story that I must tell, even though it is apropos of nothing. It concerns a friend of Ethel whose wife died soon after he retired. Not making much progress in getting a replacement, he put an ad in the newspaper. "*Retired Jewish Hematologist seeks wife.*"

Lots of women responded. After dating eight of them, he decided there must be a less fatiguing way and hit on the idea that candidates should write an essay on the topic, "*Why you should marry me.*"

Essays were received. And the winner was a forty-six-year-old blond bombshell who sent in her "essay," a full-color, full-length photo of herself in the nude. In the upper right corner, she wrote, "*I have everything you need and want.*"

Eight years later, they were still married and happy.

Back to my fellowship application.

The Fellowship of the New York Academy of Medicine was advertised throughout the city of New York. The applicants were screened down to seven, myself among them. We all assembled at the academy for the interviews. It was shocking how much the other applicants had prepared their research plans. One applicant, a doctor from Albert Einstein College of Medicine, had a gigantic tome with at least 550 pages. I didn't read it, and I am pretty sure nobody but the author read it either. But I did feel it. He let me hold it. It had heft.

The committee called me first. The chairman looked up from the papers on the table and said, "Oh, Patten. Do you have any questions?"

"No, sir."

"Well, we don't have any questions for you. You can go."

Because my interview was so short, the other candidates commiserated with me. They thought I must be out of the running. I felt sorry for them. What did they really know? Sadly, they did not know the secret workings of this world. They did not know about Irish luck. God gives the Irish tremendous luck to make up for their tremendous stupidity and to level the playing field against the Jews. It was Irish luck that led me to the men's room with Doctor Raisbeck. I had done networking in an era before the networking idea had been invented. It was I, not them, who peed next to Doctor Raisbeck, and it was I who indicated an interest in the $20,000.

Two weeks later, the Academy announced I was appointed the Memory Fellow of the New York Academy of Medicine at a yearly compensation of $20,000.

The week after that, I got the check and put the money in the stock market. Columbia gave me an office and made Mary Anne my secretary. Richard Masland, the chair of neurology, would be my supervisor and would meet me once a month to review progress or lack thereof. Doctor Masland was a wonderful person and very encouraging, but he didn't know beans about human memory. Neither did I. Nobody did.

On July 1, 1969, I started my study of human memory. Within six weeks, I had read all the books about human memory. I think there were six. And within eight weeks, I had read all the scientific papers in the world's medical literature that touched on the subject. Then… there was nothing to do.

Doctor Raisbeck was not worried. He said I should just wait for inspiration. He invited Ethel and me and Allegra and Craig to spent two weeks with him on the island he owned in the middle of the Saint Lawrence River in Canada. That would have been nice. It probably was a mistake to turn down the invitation.

Instead, I sat in my office on the second floor of the Neurological Institute of New York with my feet on the desk and read the New York Times from page one to the end. Mark Twain said that the man who doesn't read the papers is uninformed. And he said the man who reads the papers is misinformed. Thus, I was the most misinformed physician in the city. I felt fortunate to have lived in a world with so much misinformation at my fingertips. Now, with the new technology for transmitting information, we are bombarded by great quantities of small talk and frequently overwhelmed by nonsense and lots of misinformation.

The news is different these days. The reporters like to stir things up. They need to sell their product, so they try their best to make it as interesting as possible. If you believed their reports, the whole nation is on fire. None of the current news seems really important to me, and I don't like the way it is in your face 24/7. Old news was better. New news is usually bad news with lots of conflicts. Lack of conflict is considered the hallmark of all amateur journalism. If you pay any amount of mind to that Mickey Mouse stuff made King Kong sized, you might end up in a lunatic asylum or hang yourself.

Irish Luck Comes Through Again

The stagnation and lack of progress continued until one day in the middle of Christmas week, a big advertisement, a full half-page, appeared in the New York Times. In it, Harry Lorayne looked out from the page, pointing his finger directly at me with a personal message: "I can make you a memory genius."

Hot dog. Just what I needed. My haystacks weren't tied down, and I was beginning to worry about the wind. As the Memory Fellow, I was supposed to discover something to help human memory. So far, I had delivered nothing. The only thing I thought I knew about human memory was that no one knew much about it. The big question I was asking myself was the question people at a wedding ask about the groom. "We know why he is here and what he is supposed to do, but the big question is: Can he deliver?" Can I deliver? That's the question.

The short answer is yes. Harry Lorayne taught me many things about memory that were not in the medical papers or books. I adapted the Harry Lorayne methods to patient care. The techniques are now used to augment failing memories in brain-damaged patients worldwide.

In cooperation with Malcolm Conway, a commercial TWA pilot, we developed methods to train pilot memory using visual methods of thinking. The systems patented by Malcoln Conway were so efficient in training pilots that Sabena, the national airline of Belgium, purchased them for $2 million. Conway told me the North American Air Command paid him $4 million to use the systems to train the people who manage the nuclear arsenal of America. These visual systems for training memory were adapted by me and used to rehabilitate the failing verbal memories of patients who had suffered left hemisphere strokes or viral infections. Malcolm graciously excluded medical applications from his patent.

Encouraged by the new insights supplied by these two non-medical men, Conway and Lorayne, I founded the memory clinic at Columbia. The results speak for themselves. It turns out that human memory is a complex brain function that is time, content, modality, brain state, and lesion localization dependent. There is no effective limitation to human memory, and no such thing as a bad memory. There are untrained memories, yes, but no bad memories. If you like, you can read my other books about human memory and how you can dramatically increase your memory performance and look ten times smarter than you are.

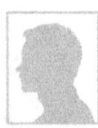

CRAIG GOES BLIND

ENCOUNTER SEVENTEEN: CRAIG GOES BLIND

◆ ◆ ◆

Craig was in the third grade in 1976, so he must have been eight years old. One Sunday, when I went up to kiss him good night and tell him I loved him, he looked at me with an inquiry face and said, "Dad, does it mean anything when you can't see out of your left eye?"

"What do you mean?"

"My left eye clouded over."

"Close your right eye and count the fingers I hold in front of your face."

"I can't see any fingers."

I called Bob Zeller, the best pediatric neurologist in Houston. "Bob, meet me in the ER. Craig lost his vision in his left eye."

There followed a frantic drive to the Texas Children's Hospital. Craig was in the back seat. Halfway there, he said, "The same thing is happening in my right eye. I can't see the moon anymore. Do you think this will affect my career as an airplane pilot?"

Bob Zeller met us at the hospital, admitted Craig, and started intravenous corticosteroids for optic neuritis. I slept in a chair in Craig's room. Either I or Ethel held him down while Bob did the spinal tap. I learned the hard way how important the medical mission is. And I learned the hard way that the last thing you can expect to get in a hospital is peace, rest, quiet, or a good night's sleep. The nurses woke us every few hours to check Craig and make sure he was still alive. They followed the orders and measured vital signs. No one expressed an interest in his vision, which was the reason we were there. We were awakened for the medicine, for a change of bed sheets (why?), for blood tests, and for examinations by what looked like medical students and residents.

The noises from outside our door got a lot worse at about six in the morning when everybody started doing things including checking pulse, blood pressure, respirations, and temperature; delivering breakfast, cleaning bedpans, moving wheelchair patients to surgery or tests. Some poor kid across the way was very unhappy and screaming his lungs out. I hoped he would be OK.

Suddenly, I realized that hospitals are in control and the patient is not. In my opinion, greater care should be paid to the comfort of the patient. Poor Craig had to dress in one of those hideous hospital gowns that opens in the back exposing his ass. That was not necessary. The hospital gown has an obsolete design, probably a century old. It provides neither warmth nor modesty. It should have gone the way of rubber baby pants for children. Craig had to stay in bed except to go to the bathroom. That was not necessary. Thank God, he had, according to the nurses, "bathroom privileges." Fancy that!

His private room was small and extra cold from too much air conditioning. The place was nearly monochromatic without any pictures or decorations—in brief, a very boring environment. The window overlooked Fannin Street, and most of the time, except for the wee hours of the morning, the street was feverish. We had no curtains, so we couldn't shut out the street lights or tone down the noise.

I had a crazy idea. We would be better off in a hotel room. I could give Craig the intravenous medicine, and we both would get adequate rest, and the room would look more commodious. The serenity would be delicious, and the cost of a hotel room to the normal ordinary patient (we were getting a free ride because of my status) would be far less than a hospital room, probably much less. My 2023 stay in the PAM (post acute medicine) hospital in Webster, Texas, cost Medicare A over $6,000 a day, physician fees, physical medicine fees, and occupational medicine fees not included. I don't care what anyone says, for Medicare to pay $6,000 a day is outrageous. Checking today, March 27, 2025, I find the famous luxury Plaza Hotel on Fifth Avenue, Manhattan, offers a full-service room for two people for $1,195 a day. How come a rehab hospital charges much more than a luxury hotel? For what Medicare and I paid to PAM for a five-day stay, my wife and I could have stayed in luxury at the Plaza Hotel for 27 days.

But somehow despite the problems, I thought it was best for us to stay in the sheltering arms of the Texas Children's Hospital. At the moment, this is where we should be. The hospital is the right place for the very sick. No question about it. I couldn't think of any place where things would likely go better for Craig.

Here's an idea: During their training, doctors and nurses should be required to strip naked, put on a hospital gown, stay in bed for a week, eat hospital food, get their sleep interrupted every four hours for vital signs, and so forth. Then they might be more sympathetic to the plight of the patients. Then someone might do something to change the routines. My same idea should be vigorously applied to hospital administrators—only they should stay longer, and not in a private room. Let the administrators suffer a semiprivate room, where the noise and the bother would be at least double and sometimes much more than double if the roommate were very sick.

Bob Zeller was one of my junior residents when I was chief resident at the Neurological Institute of New York. Then, I was in command, and Bob was just another order taker. Here he was in charge. And I did not feel demoted or envious. Nope. No resentment whatsoever, just gratitude. Bob was now like a god. Craig and I waited for Bob to round in the afternoons. We hung on every word he said, and we appreciated his caring for us as friends and not as a stranger. Bob had an upbeat, optimistic approach to the problem and made Craig and me feel comfortable about the prognosis. Hope is extremely important to patients, and it certainly was to me, hoping Craig would see again. Close your eyes and imagine what it would be like to be blind. No fun. Blindness would have an adverse effect on Craig's ambition to be an airplane pilot, as the blind can't be licensed to fly.

Almost every day, as a doctor, I made decisions that had an impact on a patient's life. Sometimes these decisions involved life or death. I always tried to do my best most of the time, but I am human. At times, there were alternative paths that I didn't consider or know about. On rare occasions, I strayed and actually made the wrong diagnosis and sent the patient to the wrong operation. One patient had myotonic dystrophy, and I thought he had myasthenia gravis. He had a thymectomy, and that had no beneficial effect. Eventually, the correct diagnosis was obvious, and I told the patient I was heartily sorry. Confession is good for the soul. When you discover a mistake that you made, it is better to admit it. Don't try to stone wall. Fortunately, that patient and his wife were sympathetic and understood. But they and I have to live with that wrong decision.

The other mistake that I think I may have made was probably more serious, as that patient is no longer with us. He probably had a treatable disease, and I misdiagnosed his treatable disease as something always fatal. I told his story in my *Maverick* book, but I will tell it again for those of you who missed it or who forgot it.

He was a 29-year-old petroleum geologist with a Ph.D. He did lots of field work doing seismographic analysis to discover oil deposits. In the field, he slept in a tent and, on multiple occasions, he was bitten by ticks, bitten many times by deer ticks.

About six months prior to the time he came to the clinic, he had trouble walking over uneven ground and stumbled and fell several times. Eventually, he developed foot drops and weakness of his arms and legs. There was no rash, no fever, no swollen joints, and no enlarged lymph nodes. About two weeks prior to the office visit, he had trouble swallowing and noticed weakness of both sides of his face. His neurologist in Tyler, Texas, thought George had motor neuron disease and sent him to me for a second opinion.

General physical exam was normal. Neurologically, he was weak with grips of 18 pounds (normal for a man his age is 86). Upper and lower extremity muscles were small, and he had to use two Canada crutches (special crutches affixed to his forearms) to walk. Sensory testing was normal to pin, vibration, soft touch, and position sense. Thus, he had motor system weakness with normal sensation, the hallmarks of motor neuron disease.

All the blood tests for the usual collection of autoimmune diseases were normal. The nerve conduction times were normal. Needle electromyography showed signs of denervation. Muscle biopsy showed small angular type I and type 2 muscle fibers. Skeletal muscle has two main fiber types: the slow oxidative fibers, called type 1, and the fast glycolytic fibers, called type 2. Both fiber types were therefore affected in his case. No inflammation was seen. The nerve biopsy showed loss of myelinated and unmyelinated fibers and loss of axons. Small patches of inflammatory cells were seen, mainly lymphocytes, so the inflammation was chronic and not acute. The spinal tap was most revealing. Spinal fluid was completely normal except for three oligoclonal bands. Oligoclonal bands usually indicate that antibodies are being produced in the nervous system. Antibodies—against what? Thus, he had an immune reaction to something. I guessed he was producing antibodies against his own nervous system tissue, and I guessed that that was making him sick. If that guess were correct, he might respond to immune suppression treatment.

Not knowing what to do, I kept him in the hospital and went to the library to do some research on the issues.

Yes, in the Golden Age of Medicine, doctors actually went to the library to research the issues related to patient care, looking for answers.

I hoped more information and some serious thinking might help. Meanwhile, George stayed in the hospital.

Three days later, waiting for me in my office was Amber (not her real name), the night nurse on Jones nine, the neurology service at the Methodist Hospital.

"Amber, what the hell is wrong. You look terrible."

"Doctor Patten, I am terrible. I did a terrible thing last night. I will resign my position at Methodist and seek psychiatric care."

"Would you like some tea or a cappuccino? I have a machine here to entertain the students and residents, but nurses can drink coffee too."

Amber shakes her head no and slumps down in my office blue leather couch.

"You know that geologist patient?"

"George?"

"Yes, George. Last night, he looked so miserable when I made rounds, I decided to cheer him up by giving him sex. I know it was unprofessional in the extreme. Sorry."

"You had sexual intercourse with George in his room in the hospital?"

"Yes, last night, about 2 a.m." Amber bows her head and wipes her eyes.

"How was it?"

"Very weak. Lots of trouble getting it up. I finally got him up with my mouth. I had to get on top and pump, and pump and pump, but I finally got him off."

"Do you want my advice?"

"I already decided to report myself to the nursing board. They will take away my license. I know that. Is that what you are driving at?"

"No, Amber. Are you kidding? You are not a good nurse. You are a great nurse. Stay on the job. Just forget it. And don't tell anyone what happened. Go thy way and sin no more."

"You're quoting Jesus from the Bible."

I nodded and smiled. Jesus often had excellent advice. Hell, Amber was just helping my patient by being compassionate. It sounded like the sex was consensual.

What would you do, dear reader? Report Amber or let it slide?

Amber continued on the job, and George continued going downhill.

Every Thursday, I made rounds by myself. On other days, I was surrounded by interns and medical students. Thursdays gave me the chance to talk to the patients directly and find out what made them tick. That evening, I made rounds on George.

"Doctor Patten, the nursing service here is super. I especially want to commend Amber for her excellent service. She is so sweet and so caring and so kind and so wonderful."

"I'll let her know."

Result: Steroid treatment didn't work. George went downhill. He refused a respirator and died at home. There was no autopsy, although I asked for one and routinely ask for an autopsy. The dead can teach us a great deal. Always get the autopsy if you or a loved one dies. The dead feel no pain. Autopsy is the best way to find out why someone died. I bet at least in a quarter of cases the autopsy shows conditions that were not diagnosed during life, some of which would have been curable. Even the best doctors are expected to be wrong some of the time. But autopsy is not a panacea or a cure-all. I have assisted at two autopsies on my own patients where the cause of death couldn't be determined. The use of modern techniques has not eliminated the need for good clinical judgment. In my view, the new breed of doctors over-relies on tests and thereby gets a false sense of security, which can lead to some gigantic errors and missed diagnoses.

Back To George the Geologist and His Case

Ten years later, at 2:35 in the morning, I woke up in a cold sweat. In my dream, I realized George had Lyme disease. He should have been treated with antibiotics. I completely blew the diagnosis, and that is why George descended into dusty death.

Lyme disease, caused by a bacterium, Borrelia burgdorferi, and spread by deer ticks, can result in serious nervous system disease like the one George had. The other possibility was tick-borne Ehrlichiosis. But George didn't have the flu-like symptoms that go with that disease. No fever, no chills meant no Ehrlichiosis. The oligoclonal bands in George's spinal fluid were probably antibodies directed against the Lyme agent and not directed against George's nervous system. On the other hand, patients with Lyme do sometimes develop autoimmune disease and require dual treatments, one for the Lyme bacterium and one for the infection-induced autoantibodies. I should have tested for Lyme disease, but I didn't even think of Lyme disease at the time.

Ugh! I missed the even bigger picture that George did have motor neuron disease, and that motor neuron disease can be caused by an infectious agent. My thinking was too conventional, too narrow. George, with his pure motor signs and progressive downhill course, could have been easily considered as a case of motor neuron disease. Because of George's case, I must force myself in ways that are counterintuitive. Such reasoning is usually wrong, but sometimes can result in a major breakthrough. Come to think on it, I have done many consultations on patients with AIDS who had all of the signs and symptoms of motor neuron disease but who recovered after treatment. Could it be that some cases of ALS are due to an infectious agent? Behind closed doors, we do wonder why a number of neurologists who specialize in taking care of ALS patients come down with and have died of ALS.

The point is that doctors make mistakes. The doctor who says he never makes mistakes is a liar and a dangerous doctor.

Yes, doctors make mistakes. But now Craig and I are in the Texas Children's Hospital. And now I am looking at things from a different point of view. Craig is the patient, and I am the worried father. I don't want any mistakes and I don't want Bob to make a wrong call or depend on statistics. I want the right medicine at the right dose by the right route for the right diagnosis. I want certain restoration of Craig's vision and will settle for nothing less.

The treatment worked.

Craig recovered his vision. He didn't become an airplane pilot, but he did get a Ph.D. in biophysics and has done important scientific work related to the neurophysiology of the brain.

Conclusion: Craig and I suffered but we were still patients in the golden age. We were met at the ER by our doctor; there were no forms and no questions about insurance or payment, and we were admitted to the Texas Children's Hospital without delay. Despite the hardships, the benefit was enormous: Craig got his vision back.

I never got a bill from the hospital or from Bob. That probably had to do with the fact that I was an attending neurologist on the hospital staff and someone somewhere felt sorry for me. Of course, I never expected a bill from Bob, and I am sure it never crossed his mind to send one. In that era, physicians did not bill physicians or their family. I took care of a fair number of doctors and their families, and I never sent a bill. Never. I did graciously accept presents, but never billed a physician or their family.

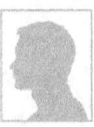

NOW WE PAUSE FOR A STRANGE INTERLUDE

NOW WE PAUSE FOR A STRANGE INTERLUDE

◆ ◆ ◆

This section divides part one from part two of this book, separating the stories of the encounters during the golden age of medicine from the more recent bronze era encounters.

Compare and contrast was the old high school suggestion to consider in your creative writing. Before we can compare and contrast, we might profit from a discussion of the types of medicine. That way, we would position ourselves to make reasonable judgments about what is good and what is not so good. It pays to know what you are thinking and talking about.

Disquisition on the Types of Medicine

First question: What are the types of medicine?

Answer: Medicine is a complex and vast subject that is so deep that no single person, including myself, knows more than a small part of it. In my view, there are two broad types of medicine:

The real and the fake. We will look at the real first, which I divide into three parts:

The Sacred Trinity of Real Medicine

1. Scientific Medicine

2. Patchwork Medicine—also known as technological medicine

3. Emphatic Medicine.

Each of these is valid in its own way and has pluses and minuses attached. Fake medicine has so many parts that they are too numerous to count. Later on, I will merely cover some amazing examples of fake medicine for your amusement and interest. Meanwhile, let's start with the real.

1. Real Medicine, Also Known as Scientific Medicine

Real medicine is scientific medicine and is effective in the extreme. It has saved millions of lives and trillions of dollars. The key feature of real medicine is the fairly complete understanding of the cause of the disease and the use of a remedy that is effective in the extreme in removing the cause. Numerous examples exist.

Polio was epidemic when I was a boy, and we feared it as we feared the plague. Kids were dying of the disease, and others were disabled, some unable to walk, and some unable to breathe. Hospitals were filled with victims, and special care facilities were established. Many iron lungs were needed to keep some victims alive. Picture for a moment the terror of being a kid sick with polio and isolated for weeks or months in an iron lung. The horror!

Massive amounts of time, energy, and money went into nursing care and nutrition care, and life support care. Many silly arguments occurred among nurses and doctors about what to do. You don't remember, but I do remember Sister Kenny and the costs of all those institutes for rehabilitation and all those ceremoniously applied hot packs. Should the paralyzed limb be passively exercised or totally immobilized? Would intramuscular gamma globulin help prevent the illness? What foods would help? What foods would hurt? How about naps? My mother insisted that my brother and I take a nap every afternoon to strengthen our resistance. Of course, I can't say we ever fell asleep. Instead, we played in the enclosed bedroom pretending to nap until Mom came to supposedly wake us up.

You get the picture. Most of the discussion about how to treat polio was pointless, just throwing sand against the tide or rowing upstream. The disease, polio, was too strong an enemy for all available measures. The treatments were supportive, and the hope was that the victims would recover, and many did, some didn't. Some of those who recovered had residual muscle atrophy and weakness lasting a lifetime. Their diagnosis was infantile paralysis, and later on, some developed the post-polio syndrome, in which the muscle paralysis gradually worsened even though the acute polio was over and the virus was no longer around.

Consider this: The tremendous costs of the polio epidemic against the enormous benefit of the vaccine. Think about how shocked I am to hear supposedly reasonable people like Robert F. Kennedy. Jr. speak against vaccination. No matter what he thinks or says, the evidence proves the polio vaccine is safe and effective. The evidence for its safety and effectiveness is beyond reasonable question. Polio vaccination is an example of scientific medicine at its best. It is scientific and effective, and relatively cheap compared to the cost of caring for the disease itself.

Another example: Smallpox. George Washington visited Barbados with his brother Lawrence in 1751. Two weeks later, George came down with smallpox. Although it was a relatively mild case, George was bedridden for weeks, rocked by high fever and chills, severe body aches, and the usual telltale rash. Mortality in the era was 30% and many victims were scarred for life. Washington survived with a few scars, and he never forgot the ordeal of being sick with smallpox.

As commander of the Continental Army, Washington had his men vaccinated against the disease, and this may have been a major factor in keeping his soldiers smallpox-free and able to fight. The actual vaccination was a lot different from the current smallpox vaccine, which is innocuous. In that era, immunization was by variolization. A small amount of pus from a patient with smallpox was rubbed into an open wound of a healthy person, resulting in the recipient's milder case of smallpox and subsequent permanent immunity. Massive epidemics of smallpox were the rule in Boston during colonial times, and thousands died of the disease. But no person vaccinated got the disease. Variolization was that effective. Now, due to scientific medicine, smallpox is a thing of the past. It amazes me, how little the public appreciates this remission from this terrible scourge. It is an example of scientific medicine at its best. It is scientific and effective, and relatively cheap compared to the cost of caring for the disease itself.

Next example:

A hoarse and shaky voice: "I want to speak to the doctor."

"Yuh—yuh—'S the doctor speaking."

"This is Henry Novak, four miles northeast, on the Leopolis road. My little girl, Mary, she has a terrible sore throat. I think maybe it is croup and she looks awful and—Could you come right away?"

"You bet. Be right there."

It was forty minutes from the time of the telephone call when he rushed into a furrowed driveway and saw on the doorstep, against the lamplight, a stooped man who called, "The Doctor? This is Novak."

He found the child in a newly finished bedroom of white plastered walls and pale varnished pine. Only an iron bed, a straight chair, a chromo of Saint Anne (mother of Mary and grandmother of Jesus), and a shadeless hand-lamp on a rickety stand broke the staring shininess of the apartment, a recent extension of the farmhouse. A heavy-shouldered woman was kneeling by the bed.

As she lifted her wet, red face, Novak urged: "Don't cry now; he's here."

And to the doctor: "The little one is pretty bad, but we've done all we could for her. Last night and tonight we steamed her throat, and we put her here in our own bedroom."

Mary was a child of seven or eight. Her fingertips and lips were blue, but her face had no flush. In the effort to expel her breath, she writhed into terrible knots, then coughed up saliva dotted with greyish specks.

The doctor felt helpless without the equipment of the hospital and the nurses and a senior doctor's advice. Suddenly he had a profound respect for the lone country doctor which he now was. What to do? He had to make a decision.

Operate? Or get diphtheria antitoxin? It was too late for anything short of antitoxin or tracheotomy.

The child was still alive when he got back with the antitoxin. Swiftly and smoothly, he made the intravenous injection and stood expectant.

Mary choked in the labor of expelling her breath. There was a gurgle, a struggle in which her face turned blue-black, and she was still. Slowly, they knew she was gone.

Apologies to Sinclair Lewis and his masterpiece of American literature (now out of copyright), *Arrowsmith*. Yep, that's the way the kids died of diphtheria. And that is the way my Aunt Mary Patten died in a small bedroom of the Patten family apartment in Astoria. She aspirated the diphtheria membrane and choked to death. Who would wish this torture on anybody, much less a child? And yet there are fools out there in ga-ga land who would speak against a vaccination that is effective in the extreme. Where are the cases of diphtheria now? You guessed it: They are gone with the wind. There are none. There are none among the vaccinated. The same holds for many of the serious childhood illnesses that are now preventable by the application of scientific medicine.

Now hear this! Things can and do go wrong when fools do not permit their children to get vaccinated. The current 661 cases of measles now raging in the backwater sections of Texas and New Mexico are a startling example. So far, there has been lots of morbidity but only three deaths.

Side Bar About Diphtheria Showing How Complex Biology Can Be

Sorry! Sometimes I am just bursting to give interesting information. The real cause of diphtheria is not the diphtheria bacillus, which is harmless. The cause is the toxin produced when the bacillus is infected with a phage, a virus that infects bacteria. It is the phage that encodes the diphtheria toxin, and it is that toxin that produces the disease. So, a child with the disease diphtheria is a victim of a viral infection, but not of the virus itself. It is the bacteria that have the viral infection, and the human gets sick as a sort of innocent bystander. Biology! Whew! Biology is truly amazing and much more complex than most people imagine, and probably much more complex than we can imagine.

Stop now. Pretend you are a scientist and need to make a vaccine to prevent death from diphtheria. What should be the target of your vaccine: The bacillus or the toxin?

The toxin, of course. The same for tetanus. Give yourself a pat on the back if you got the answer right.

It amazes me, how little this remission from these terrible scourges is appreciated by the public. It is an example of scientific medicine at its best. It is scientific and effective and relatively cheap compared to the cost of caring for the disease itself.

Other examples of scientific medicine:

Public health: This is a major scientific field that has saved many lives and eliminated much suffering. For example, none of our treatments for late-stage lung cancer have reduced mortality by nearly as much as the worldwide reduction in smoking, thanks in part to the smoking bans. Promotion of exercise has done much to prolong lifespans and preserve cognitive and physical function. Pure water and food give us gigantic health benefits as does the flush toilet and modern sewer systems. Environmental protection is particularly important because of the health consequences of air pollution. There are places on our planet (known in the medical literature as "blue zones") where people live longer than average. Those places do not share a common climate or geography, but they do have common elements that prolong life. In general, those places (Okinawa, Loma Linda) have no air pollution. From the air we breathe to the water we drink, our well-being is directly linked to our ecosystems. The current tendency in America to dismantle environmental protections in favor of financial interests is unscientific and deplorable.

More examples of scientific medicine:

When properly applied, antibiotics have been amazingly lifesaving. The trick is to identify exactly the organism causing the disease and its sensitivity to the appropriate antibiotic. Then, the antibiotic is given to the right patient at the right time, by the right route, with the right dose, for the right amount of time. Remarkable cures are expected from this approach and are commonplace.

Think about typhoid fever. If a case of typhoid fever had to be managed today by the best methods of 1941, when I was born, the expense would be staggering. There would be about fifty days of misery in a hospital, much pain and suffering, with the most demanding 24/7 nursing care, daily laboratory monitoring with management of fluid and electrolytes, tricky nutritional provisions, and surgical intervention for the occasional abdominal catastrophe. The dollar cost, according to Doctor Lewis Thomas's conservative estimate, was $10,000, which in today's dollars would be $230,412. Compare that cost with the current cost of a bottle of chloramphenicol ($57.04) and a day or two of fever.

Another example: The capacity to effectively deal with syphilis and tuberculosis is a gigantic milestone in human achievement, even though full use of these treatments has not yet occurred for a large segment of the world's population.

By the way, if you think the eradication of tuberculosis is not such a big deal. Think again. Poor Chopin struggled with fever, terrible weakness and fatigue, night sweats, while composing the preludes. How much more beautiful music the world would have had if he had not died of T.B. at age 39.

Yours truly and another assistant physician, in 1966, took care of ward G3H3 at the New York Hospital, Cornell Medical Center. We had 54 patients, all of whom had T.B. except one young man who had acute leukemia. The morbidity of T.B. was terrible, with patients who had the pulmonary form, and even worse among the many who had systemic infections with total organ failure. There was even a child with hip arthritis from the tubercle bacillus and a pathetic 30-year-old pregnant woman who had tuberculous meningitis, which in that era was always fatal. There were two men with tuberculous sepsis, an infection of the blood. They arrested (that is, their hearts stopped) almost at the same time. I tried to resuscitate one but failed and both died within ten minutes of each other. Most of my care was spent trying to improve the breathing of the patients with pulmonary involvement. Most of the measures—nasal O2, venti mask (a special mask to administer graded amounts of oxygen), and intubation (putting a tube in the windpipe and hooking it to a machine that would ventilate the patient) were temporary measures against the disease that was too strong for us. Hold your breath for as long as you can so you can appreciate how terrible it is not to be able to take a breath. Thank the fates all that is a thing of the past. The sanatoria are no longer needed. Sanatoria weren't so great anyway. Over 50% of patients who entered sanatoria died within five years. Travel to a warm climate is no longer prescribed. Surgical collapse of the lung (pneumothorax) is done to "rest" the infected lung, no longer needed. Now we have streptomycin and isoniazid, and rifampicin, sanitation, vaccination, and public health measures.

To whom do we owe the great advances in control and cure of T.B.? Lots of scientists, including Robert Koch, who identified the bacillus that causes the disease (Nobel Prize in Medicine 1905 for his work), and Selman Abraham Waksman, who proved streptomycin effective in killing the bacillus (Nobel Prize in Medicine 1952 for his work).

To whom do we owe the conquest of polio? Lots of scientists. But once it was learned from basic research that there exist three antigenic types of polio virus and that all three could be grown in tissue culture, the development of an effective vaccine was certain. So, the Nobel Prize was awarded in 1954 to John Enders, Frederick Robbins, and Thomas Weller for their work in culturing the polio virus. The production of the vaccine naturally followed and was a great accomplishment, but not as great as the basic research that made the vaccine possible.

Recently, there has been tremendous progress in the development of antivirals. Hepatitis C can now be cured. Yes, cured. The virus was completely eliminated, and the patient was completely well. That miracle has saved many a patient from the ordeal and expense of a liver transplant. And need I mention that AIDS patients now can live a normal or close to normal life span thanks to antiviral treatment. No need to remind you that untreated AIDS is fatal. Lenacapavir, the new antiviral from Gilead Sciences, is effective in the extreme as the pre-exposure prophylaxis of Human Immune Deficiency Disease and in combination with other antivirals may, sometime in the future, actually cure the disease.

Here is the point:

Really effective medicine comes as the result of a real, deep, and complete understanding of disease mechanisms.

When that kind of understanding is achieved and the results become generally available, medical treatment becomes relatively inexpensive, relatively simple, and relatively easy to deliver. It is nice to think there are so many unsolved mysteries in biology—real puzzles that need careful and detailed attention to be solved, although I wonder if we will ever find enough youths interested in such work. Most of the kids I know seem more stoked on investment banking, finance, or merchandising. And President Trump has cut the support of postgraduate students who do most of the original basic medical research.

When doctors get bogged down by incomplete knowledge of what they are dealing with, when they lack a complete understanding of the disease mechanism, and don't have a clear idea of what to do, like the situation on ward G3H3 with my T.B. patients, the deficiencies of the present health care system become conspicuous.

Some Past Faux Pas

Tonsils and adenoids that should have been left in place were removed. The operations were often justified by the claim that they were or could become foci of infection.

Enlarged thymus glands in children were treated with X-rays on the crazy theory that the enlarged gland was harmful in some unspecified way. Later in life, many of these thymuses became cancerous.

DES (diethylstilbestrol), a synthetic (man-made) form of estrogen, was given to prevent miscarriage. The daughters developed cancers of the genital tract.

Thalidomide was given to help pregnant women with morning sickness, insomnia, and nervousness. Over 10,000 kids were born with a wide range of defects in the eyes, heart, including phocomelia, no arms, just hands coming right off the shoulders.

Appetite suppressants to lose weight resulted in cataracts.

On and on, the list seems endless.

I do not influence policy because I am just an old man on the way out. Not that I mind being on the way out or being old. There is no better time in history to be old, and I am grateful that I have lived so long because many of my friends have been denied that privilege. But if I were a policymaker, I would attach a high priority to a lot more basic research. That is the way in the long run we get full mileage out of tax dollars. To solve the cancer problem, for instance, we need to know a hell of a lot more about the physiology of the cancer cell and how to correct and redirect that problematic biology. That knowledge about cancer will require time and energy to discover. And, oh, yes, money too. And lots of graduate students.

Right now, billions are being spent planning a visit to Mars. President Trump said he wants to plant an American flag there.

<u>Why colonize Mars when we are so busy wrecking our own planet?</u>

The current estimate, according to Science magazine on January 10, 2025, is $4 billion. We have, in my view, many more problems here on earth that are worth that kind of investment. In fact, the only reason I can see to go to Mars is that Elvis Presley is there and has ordered a pizza and a Coke.

2. Patchwork Medicine—also known as technological medicine

At the next level down, we have what I call patchwork medicine. It has its pluses and minuses, and mainly involves what should be done after the fact. This form of medicine is an attempt to compensate for incomplete knowledge of the disease mechanism and the lack of a really effective treatment in preventing or reversing the condition. The technology is designed to ease the disease's burden and postpone death or both. Some doctors seem down on the idea of preventing death, claiming death is natural, so we should simply accept it as such. Gawande in his book *Being Mortal*, if I read him correctly, says as much. Not me! Death is the enemy.

Death is OK because it is natural. The wheels fall off that "natural" argument pretty quickly if you think about it for two minutes. Is it natural to wear shoes? Is it natural to brush your teeth? Is it natural to get vaccinated against smallpox and polio? If I have pneumonia, is it better to let the disease run its natural course or to increase the chance of survival by getting penicillin?

Death is natural, but that doesn't make it desirable or good. In general, beware the natural arguments. Feces are natural, but you would not want to eat them. Because a food or a remedy is natural doesn't necessarily make it good or desirable. Lots of non-natural things may be better. In my view, survival is the name of the game. Your personal survival, your family's survival, the survival of your friends and relatives, and the survival of our species. Natural or not natural: we must choose what works best for health and longevity.

The aim of this section of real medicine is promotion of life, especially useful life. Therefore, in my view, patchwork medicine is important and should play a major role in human survival.

We are talking here about transplants of hearts, kidneys, livers, and other organs. The public seems to think and accept these tricks as the equivalent of major break-throughs and therapeutic triumphs instead of the makeshifts they really are. This level of medicine must continue until there is a genuine scientific understanding of the mechanisms involved in the disease in question. Take idiopathic pulmonary fibrosis, for instance. This is a chronic, irreversible, and ultimately fatal disease characterized by a progressive decline in lung function. Medical textbooks say the cause is "idiopathic cryptogenic fibrosing alveolitis." The very name denotes our ignorance of the cause of the fibrosis of the lungs. This disease is idiopathic, mean-ing the cause is not known. The pathology itself is labelled "cryptogenic," mean-ing obscurely caused. The lack of a real understanding of the cause and how to reverse it entails falling back on the patchwork treatment called a lung transplant. Like the transplants mentioned above, much time, energy, skill, and expense are involved in addition to the urgent need for (did you guess it?) a donated lung, or, even better, a donated pair of lungs. Much organization and sophistication are needed to successfully carry out this treatment and, of course, from the perspec-tive of the individual recipient patient, who is always near death from the disease, lung transplant looks like a pardon, a reprieve, a godsend. The patients and family members I have talked to view the result as a miracle. It is not a miracle of course. It is the result of the direct application of advanced technology and lots of science at the bedside and in the operating room.

According to a recent article in the New England Journal of Medicine (NEJM 391;17,1822-1836) the multidisciplinary care team for a lung transplant consists of transportation pulmonologists, transplantation surgeons, transplantation coor-dinators, pharmacists, nutritionists, pulmonary rehabilitation specialists, physical therapists, social workers, critical care specialists, endocrinologists, immunolo-gists, infectious disease experts, gastroenterologists, psychiatrists, and financial coordinators.

But wouldn't it be better, much better, in fact, to have a clear insight into the immune mechanisms operating here and to be able with some sweet antidote to reverse the process? When such a level of understanding is reached, the patchwork of lung transplant will not be much needed and will no longer pose the huge problems of logistics and ethics (who gets the treatment and who doesn't and why?).

Another major ethical problem with any patchwork treatment is tremendous cost. Who should pay and how much? When? And why?

Survival after lung transplant, as compared with other organ transplantation, remains limited at a median of 6.7 years, with little progress with respect to long-term survival outcomes over the last three decades. However, in the meanwhile, many patients have substantial improvements in quality of life, physical performance, and other patient-oriented outcomes like return to work. The main problem is CLAD, chronic lung allograft dysfunction due to bronchiolitis obliterans or RAD, the restrictive allograft dysfunction. Some unlucky patients have both complications, called CLAD mixed. Therapy for these problems is largely ineffective. More research is needed to resolve CLAD and RAD because they are almost always fatal.

By the way, the existence of CLAD proves that the chronic fibrosis of lungs is not due to a defect in the lung, but must reside elsewhere. The lung is the target of the disease process and that is proven by the fact that the lung transplant from a lung healthy doner gets the lung fibrosis that was the original reason for the transplant. Therefore, the disease process must be in the body of the recipient of the transplant.

At present, almost every treatment of heart disease is at the patch level with specialized ambulances, amply equipped intensive care units (ICU), all kinds of electronic gadgetry even if you don't have heart disease and (I know this from personal ICU experience as a patient and as a doctor) parades of professional specialists each charging hefty fees. It is a characteristic of heart technology that it expands and expands with no end in sight. There is no question that this has resulted in the extension of life for some patients. But is it really worth it on a cost-benefit analysis? The dark side of me thinks there has been an over expansion of the technology, resulting in some specialists looking for more to do. My dance partner had no clinical signs of heart disease (no angina, no shortness of breath, no pedal, foot, edema and so forth) but she had ultrasound studies of her heart and great vessels including carotids and aorta plus a thallium stress test and a cardiac catheterization, all of which proved normal. When she asked her doctor why she needed all those tests she says she was told "to prevent a heart attack or a stroke because your cholesterol is 200, which is at the upper level of normal." Total cholesterol is only slightly more relevant to cardiovascular risk than eye color. Her repeat cholesterol was 168! Ye gods, the repeat may have prevented all that testing.

When we figure out how to reverse the processes that cause heart disease, the current elaborate technology will be set aside as obsolete, just the way we no longer use whale oil or kerosene to light our homes and no longer need a buggy whip because most of us don't have a horse and carriage, and buggy whips do not speed up internal combustion engines.

Much of what is currently done for cancer (surgery, radiation, chemo) is what I consider patchwork medicine because these measures are directed at already established cancer cells, but not at the exact biological mechanisms that cause the cells to become neoplastic, that is cancer-like. Thus, cancer costs an enormous amount of money and requires continuing expansion of hospital facilities with lots of specialized doctors spending lots of time on the problems. There is no end to this progression of more and more technology in view of the present state of poor scientific knowledge of what exactly is wrong in cancer and what exactly needs to be done to correct and reverse it.

The only thing that can move us away from current partially effective patch medicine, the only thing that can move us away from our current ignorance, and toward 100% effective scientific medicine that would include a cancer cure as effective as the completely effective cure for hepatitis C—that only thing is new information, and the source of new information has to be medical and biologic research.

In part two of this book, we will review real-world encounters with patchwork medicine. The most successful patchwork in the view of most physicians is cataract surgery. Last time I checked, there were seven main types of cataracts, but only one of these is the known cause. The sunburst blue cataract of Wilson's disease is due to the deposit of copper in the lens. In theory, this cataract could be prevented by early diagnosis of Wilson's disease and the use of low-copper diets and medicines that remove copper from tissue. But that is in theory. In practice, the diagnosis is often made very late in the illness, and permanent damage to the tissues (lens, liver, cornea, muscle, nerve, central nervous system, and so forth) has already been done by toxic levels of copper and can no longer be completely reversed.

For the other six types of cataracts, our information about prevention and reversal is close to zero. Part of the reason is that the surgery is so effective and part of the reason is that cataract is considered a natural consequence of aging. Aging does seem to promote cataract formation. So what! Aging and all biologic processes are based on physical and chemical processes, so there is no a priori reason to assume cataract formation is any different. All physical and chemical processes are potentially reversible or can be inhibited or abated.

I personally have seen cataracts in a newborn child who had rubella, proving that age is not the only factor. I have seen cataracts in adolescents, particularly among those who have type I diabetes, and I have seen many cataracts associated with the corticosteroid treatments of various autoimmune diseases. And I have witnessed cataracts disappear, proving that cataracts can, under certain conditions, reverse the clouded lens to clear normal. This is certainly true of the posterior subcapsular cataracts associated with steroid use. If the steroids are stopped, the cataract may cure itself.

If we knew all in all what, in physical and chemical terms, was causing the lens to get opaque and if we knew how to reverse the process, then all cataract surgery would become as obsolete as cupping, bleeding, and purging. And there would be an enormous saving of time, energy, and costs. Last year, the estimated cost of direct care for cataract surgery in the United States was $7 billion.

Another beef: Osteoarthritis. My friends, when asked what caused their osteoarthritis and required the replacement of the damaged hip or knee joint with a fake device, reply, "Degeneration of the knee due to wear and tear and aging." That is a diversionary argument away from the realization that the real cause of the condition is not understood. In my view, the diseased joints are merely the target of the disease process, which originates somewhere else that we can't even imagine. Recent evidence proves osteoarthritis is due to a gut bacterium making a chemical that targets the cartilage in the joints. That kind of research is more likely to produce a real prevention and real cure of this common condition. To learn more, consult Science April 2025, VOL 388 ISSUE 6742, page 48 and follow.

Before we leave patchwork medicine, I wish to tell you about things that trouble my sleep. As an old-time physician who believed and still believes the clinical condition of the patient should control what happens, I am philosophically against screening for disease in healthy people. I guess we could supply care for everyone needing it if we could restrain ourselves from assuming that all 350 million Americans are in constant peril of failing health every day of their lives. The American legal system assumes us to be innocent until proven guilty. In my view, a medical system works best if it starts with the presumption that most people are healthy most of the time. The great secret I learned early in my medical career—a secret that the general public should know—is that most things get better by themselves.

My favorite treatment is no treatment at all.

Doctors and doctor families receive far less medical attention than friends or neighbors. Nevertheless, they seem a normal, generally healthy lot, with a remarkably low incidence of iatrogenic (doctor-caused) disease.

The problem is that screening takes time and money, and often finds nothing wrong. Therefore, there was a waste of time and energy. But the bigger problem is that screening may find something wrong. That something will then be a thing under investigation, with the burden of cost and time, and anxiety falling on the individual patient. Screening itself can have adverse consequences. For example, one of my colleagues, an internationally known expert in muscle disease, at age 72, married his graduate student who was 42 years younger than he. His wife was shocked that he had never had a colonoscopy, and she insisted that he have one. So, to please her, my friend had a colonoscopy. It was normal. No polyps. No cancer. No nothing. But during the procedure, the scope broke open the colon, and fecal material spilled into the abdomen. According to Healthline, this complication occurs 31 times among 100,000 colonoscopies. Severe infection followed. E.L. then spent 6 weeks in intensive care at death's door, in and out of shock, almost dying from sepsis.

Lesson: Not only was the screening negative for disease, but it itself produced a major life-threatening health problem. According to Healthline, from 2015 to 2019, colonoscopy found 35.7 cancers per 100,000 procedures. In other words, it took an average of 2,801 colonoscopies to find one cancer. According to the same source, there were, on average, 146 episodes of significant bleeding per 100,000 procedures and, as mentioned, 31 perforations. In a ~19.5-year risk follow-up of people who had 2 to 9 colonoscopies during that time period, the hazard ratio for colon cancer (HR) was 0.91, a value pretty close to HR 1, the natural incidence of colon cancer. Is that meager result worth all the preparation and trouble, and cost? Who knows? I have no clear answer. There has to be a cut-off age (about 75?) where even the detection of a premalignant polyp makes no sense because the patient is likely to die of something other than colon cancer.

It is now generally acknowledged that screening for prostate cancer detects a large number of small cancers that probably would have had no adverse effect on the man's lifespan or health. Prostate cancers are sometimes very malignant and at other times relatively benign. In other words, there are cancers with a big C and cancers with a little c. The little c cancers have been over-treated, with many men having bowel and bladder, and erectile problems from the treatment and not from the disease. It also seems to me that some kinds of breast cancer are being over-treated. Purely intraductal adenocarcinoma of the breast might be a case in point because it is probable that this type of breast cancer is unlikely to spread.

Incidental Findings

Sometimes in the course of screening or a workup for a clinical problem, another thing shows up, and that can focus attention on itself. When I developed gross bleeding from my penis, the cystoscopy showed the cause of bleeding was an abnormal artery vein connection in my bladder. But in the course of looking for other possible causes of bleeding, an ultrasound showed a one-centimeter round lesion in the right kidney. That lesion could not have been a source of bleeding into my urine. It was merely an incidental finding not related in any manner, shape, or form to my clinical problem. But it did put me on the medical merry-go-round for three years because my urologist said we had to make sure I didn't have cancer of the kidney.

So repeated tests were done to see if the kidney thing was a cancer or not. Some sonograms showed what appeared to be a cyst; sometimes the sonograms showed the lesion was not there, and the kidney was normal. Kidney, ureter, and bladder x-rays failed to show the kidney lesion that the ultrasound detected. So, for three years full of uncertainty, I spent lots of time waiting for the tests to be done, and then waiting for the test results, and then waiting for the doctor's advice about the tests and what to do next. This elusive search for a kidney cancer in myself reminds me of the actual accidental finding of a kidney cancer in one of my patients.

She had severe myasthenia gravis, a very serious disease wherein muscles become very weak, sometimes preventing the patient from breathing. Her condition came under control after much hard work. By accident, an X-ray was taken of the patient's abdomen when only a chest X-ray was ordered. The accidental abdominal X-ray showed what appeared to be a cancer of the kidney. Needle biopsy of the tumor proved it was a clear cell carcinoma of the kidney. Now the question was what to do. What would you do, dear reader? Operate to remove the kidney to prevent malignant spread, or not operate? The problem with the operation would be that the patient would have to undergo anesthesia and surgery, which for a myasthenic would be quite risky. Operation would also leave her with only one kidney and thus reduce her defense against kidney disease by half.

I pause for reply.

Stop and think: What would you do? How should this clear cell cancer of the kidney be treated? The standard care and the usual treatment are surgical removal of the involved kidney, leaving the patient with only one remaining kidney and a big medical bill.

What's your view? Write it down so we know exactly where you stand on how this incidentally detected kidney cancer should be treated. If you can, give reasons for your opinion and predict what will happen to this patient if the kidney cancer is not removed.

My view: This is what doctors call an incidentaloma. A cancer incidentally discovered. It is causing no problems for the patient except the anxiety engendered by knowing she has a definite diagnosis of kidney cancer. The prognosis of tumors discovered incidentally is usually much better than that of cancers discovered because they are causing clinical signs or symptoms or both.

Actual management:

Discretion is the better part of valor. So, my patient and I decided we would just watch and wait and see what kind of cancer this might be. Is it a big C CANCER or a little c cancer? Is it biologically malignant or not? Histologically, this is a cancer. Under the microscope, the pathologist and I saw it had all of the hallmarks of cancer, so the histological diagnosis of cancer is beyond doubt and fully confirmed.

Usually, there is a tight connection between the histological diagnosis of cancer and the actual clinical features and progression of the malignancy. But usually means that sometimes there is not a direct correlation between the pathological appearance of the cancer and the biological activity of the cancer. In other words, a cancer can look malignant under the microscope but actually be biologically benign. In my own practice, I have seen that can be true, and I have seen just the opposite can also be true: A histologically benign thymic tumor was actually biologically malignant and killed my patient. At autopsy, the tumor still looked histologically benign, even though it had spread over most of the thorax and choked the great vessels and the lungs, and invaded the heart. That tumor looked benign under the microscope but was actually biologically malignant.

Strictly speaking, the tissue diagnosis of cancer is on the way out as a single test of the biology of cancer. Cell markers and the study of special metabolic requirements of some cancers have led to amazing cures that approach the kind of real scientific medicine cures seen in infectious disease. More detailed studies of individual cancers have shown that cancer biology is complex in the extreme. The more we understand cancer's biology, chemistry, and biophysics, the more power we will have over this dread disease.

Last time I checked, there were six different biological types of malignant melanoma, some of which have a unique metabolism that makes them amenable to spectacular cure, and yet each looks pretty much the same under the microscope, and each will be reported out of routine pathological examination as malignant melanoma.

Only time will tell in this case of a patient with histologically proven cancer whether the cancer is biologically malignant or not. But if we do not operate on the patient's cancer, are we not risking the spread of the cancer, leading to a cancer death in the future? Aye, there's the rub. The future is unknown and contingent on many factors, some of which are known and some of which are unknown. One man bragged to me that the doctors opened his abdomen to remove a cancer of the pancreas and quickly closed. The patient and family were told the situation was hopeless and death would be likely in less than six months. And here he was, six years later, and completely well. I love checking stories like this. It turns out that the diagnosis before exploratory operation was cancer of the pancreas, and the family and patient were told of the poor prognosis. Nevertheless, they wanted to know for sure and wanted the surgeon to open and see.

GUESS WHAT! THE DIAGNOSIS WAS NO CANCER FOUND. THE PATIENT HAD PANCREATITIS.

Result in my myasthenic patient who really did have kidney cancer: Thirty years later, my patient with biopsy-proven cancer of the kidney is entirely well. The histologically proven cancer has not changed one bit. It is the same size, shape, and is in the same location, and there has been no spread or growth.

Lesson: Under some circumstances, even a definite tissue diagnosis of malignancy doesn't necessarily mean treatment is needed.

In this case, keeping our hands in our pockets and doing nothing (for a good reason: to save her the risk of operation) but observation saved the patient a needless operation and saved her kidney from removal. She did have the inconvenience of yearly studies of the cancer to make sure it was not growing. But those yearly checks saved her the trouble and expense of operation and assured her that all was well.

While we are on the topic, here is another thing that bothers me: Some unnecessary procedures are done on patients who are doomed to die very soon. My neighbor and great friend, Vince Johnson, had metastatic cancer of the lung. He could find no doctor willing to work on his case because, frankly, his lung cancer was hopeless. Nevertheless, a Mohs surgery (a type of surgery with repeated checks of the removed tissue to make sure all the skin cancer was removed) was done on a skin cancer on his bald scalp. The surgery required sitting time and repeated surgery, followed by histologic examination of the removed tissue to make sure there was no cancer of the skin at the surgical margins. Vince spent about four hours getting his little skin cancer completely removed. The surgical wound was still oozing fluid two weeks later. What was all this for? It was like rearranging the deck chairs on the Titanic, something to do that would have no effect on the major problem or the outcome. There was no way the skin cancer was going to have any clinical effect on Vince's life or health. He was already doomed to die of lung cancer, and he could have better spent his time planning his funeral or saying goodbye to his son, Blake.

Six weeks after the complete removal of a small skin cancer, Vince died of a complication of lung cancer. The removal of the skin cancer was, in my opinion, a complete waste of time and energy for Vince, but it did financially benefit the dermatologist who did the surgery.

Lesson: A sense of balance and proportion should be applied to each and every medical problem. Avoid minoring the major problem and majoring the minor problem. In Vince's case, the skin cancer was a minor problem that was trivial and should have been left alone. In other words, majoring in the minor was wrong. The lung cancer was the major problem, unfortunately, beyond repair.

Let's Talk About Tests

The public in general has a rather naïve attitude toward tests. In the old days, medical students and interns had our own laboratories. As an intern, if I ordered a blood gas determination on my patient, I would have to draw the arterial sample, take it to the intern's laboratory, and do the test myself. This was an excellent experience that taught me that test results can vary even when I, a trained chemist, was doing the measurements. Usually, I would do three quantitative analyses, and guess what? I would get three different values. Which one is the real value? Hard to say.

Modern commercial laboratories have the same problem. If I draw three samples from the same patient at the same time and send them to three different laboratories, I usually get back three different results. This happens even if the samples are sent to the same laboratory.

The problem is what physicists know for sure: It is impossible to measure any-thing accurately and precisely. Every measurement is more or less approximate.

In the hands of the inexperienced physician, false results can lead to unnecessary treatment or to no treatment for a missed diagnosis.

My patient with obvious copper storage disease was reported to have a normal ceruloplasmin. Talking to the technician who did the test revealed that she did the test several times and came up with a zero, that is, no ceruloplasmin. That is the expected result and is almost diagnostic of the copper storage disease. But she had never seen a zero on this test before, so she felt she might have done the test wrong, so she just wrote down a normal number. We fired her, of course. Another tech reported out an anti-nuclear antibody test as normal in a patient with severe lupus. The tech said he did the test many times and kept coming out 25,000 (normal is below 25), so he figured he did the test wrong and just reported out a normal value. We fired him, too.

After the detailed neurological exam, the neurologist proved to me that I had a combined system disease due to B12 deficiency. She said she didn't care that the lab reported a normal B12 level for me. Repeat B12 test in a different laboratory subsequently confirmed her diagnosis. The clinical response I had to the B12 in-jections was excellent; the cerebellar tremor disappeared, my leg nerves recovered, my tap dancing improved, and so forth—all that confirmed the clinical diagnosis and proved the first laboratory B12 test was wrong. What bothered me is that several physicians told me it was impossible for me to be B12 deficient in view of the first test result that came back normal. It hadn't even crossed their minds that the original lab was wrong and the neurologist was right.

Keep in mind that tests are not necessarily innocuous. Doctors love to do them; it makes medicine seem scientific. Because a missed diagnosis can mean a lawsuit, there is a tendency to overtest as part of what is called defensive medicine. I guess that is understandable. But it is not understandable why a patient in the hospital should have a chest X-ray every day and multiple complete blood counts every day.

In the old days, SBE (subacute bacterial endocarditis, an infection of a heart valve) was an incurable disease. Because there was no effective treatment, the arguments on rounds revolved around how many aspirins should be given or whether the windows should be open or closed. Since nothing could be done to really stop the disease, the attendings did what they could do—namely, ordered more and more tests.

<u>Another thing to keep in mind: If you see it, you believe it. If you don't see it, you don't know. It could still be there, but you missed it or used the wrong diagnosis tool.</u>

If I use a telescope and report no bacteria seen, it doesn't mean there are no bacteria. A microscope is the tool to see bacteria. Thus, a negative test means next to nothing. And many negative tests can mean nothing. One of my patients had 87 negative blood cultures while she was alive because I suspected SBE as the cause of her heart murmur and fever. I even treated her with antibiotics on the hunch she had SBE despite the negative blood cultures. Autopsy proved she had SBE despite all those negative cultures. Why the bug didn't grow in lab blood cultures but did grow at autopsy was never explained. Why she failed to respond to massive intravenous doses of antibiotics is also a puzzle.

Early in my career, I also learned not to trust the X-ray reports. All films on my patients were personally reviewed by me to ensure accuracy. There have been X-rays read as cancer of the colon when what was seen was just a piece of stool. Recently, a friend asked me to review a brain CAT scan on her daughter, who had severe headaches. The scan had been read by a neuroradiologist as normal when it showed a colloid cyst of the third ventricle obstructing the aqueduct of Sylvius and producing severe hydrocephalus. The daughter needed emergency decompression to prevent brain stem compression, and she got it just in time. Chest x-rays, in my experience, are often misread, leading to a missed diagnosis. Studies have shown that radiologists will disagree about 30% of the time on what a chest X-ray shows. I have known good pathologists disagree on whether a biopsy is benign or malignant. That's hell for the patient.

In Houston, fair city, we had three physicians who used to read muscle biopsies, myself and two others. After I read a biopsy, I could predict with almost 92% accuracy what the other two would say. Who was right? Me, of course. Actually, I was probably more right because I knew the patient's history and physical findings and was in a better position to align the reading with the clinical picture.

Artificial Intelligence (AI) may improve things, but I doubt it. The term artificial intelligence is misleading. It is different from human intelligence, very different. A kid only needs to see a cat once before they can identify all cats in the future. Artificial intelligence needs to see millions of cat pictures (and loads of electricity) before it can work well. And artificial intelligence is subject to adversarial attacks. Put only a few extraneous pixels in the picture, and artificial intelligence gets things hopelessly wrong. Recently, I took a picture of a large cauliflower and a picture of a smaller cauliflower, both from my garden. Artificial intelligence identified the separated vegetables correctly, but when I showed a picture of the two together with the small one touching the big, artificial intelligence became hopelessly confused and identified nothing. To the human eye, there was no problem. The picture just shows two cauliflowers next to each other.

Last but not least, we come to the third type of medicine.

Did you remember what one and two were?

1. One was scientific medicine and

2. Two was patchwork medicine.

3. The third is Emphatic medicine or compassionate medicine.

Emphatic Medicine

Emphatic medicine is medicine in which it is not possible to measure exactly the effect on the natural course of the disease or the eventual outcome. A great deal of time and money is spent on this type of medicine, and it is highly valued by doctors and patients. Some call this type of medicine "supportive medicine" or "supportive therapy." It is important in tiding patients through or over diseases that are not quite understood. This is what is meant by caring for or standing by or holding hands. In my view, it is indispensable and a featured component of all successful medical practices. Because it is not directed at the underlying cause of the disease, compassionate medicine takes up a good part of the doctor's time explaining things, providing comfort and reassurance, and hope. This is the form of medicine I discussed when I talked about Doctor Lanza. He gives assurance to people who fear they have contracted a lethal disease when they are quite healthy or will soon be fully recovered and quite healthy. He knew our family, and we knew him. This was the kind of medicine that the old-time doctors did at the bedside while waiting for the pneumonia crisis, the peak of the disease, to occur. They patiently watched the patient who had meningitis, diphtheria, polio, and all the rest of the infectious diseases of which we now have pretty good control.

This is the medicine that physicians must now do for patients with intractable conditions like cancer, severe arthritis, stroke, chronic obstructive lung disease, kidney failure, and so forth. I can think of at least 186 diseases that require this kind of help and support. This is needed because of the absence of an effective treatment. My view is that a large amount of mental health care is also this type of medicine, supportive but not really getting to the cause of the problem, and certainly not curing it.

The cost of this type of medicine is high, and getting higher. It requires a great deal of professional time and great understanding of the patient. Few physicians can do it effectively, and many do not want to do it because the direct financial rewards are slim.

There are few codes for compassionate care, and the pay is low. In modern medicine, what is not paid for is often neglected, not supported, and therefore not done.

Emphatic care requires that the doctor understand and relate to the patient as a person. On rounds, I do not want to hear about the kid in room 503 with a brain tumor. I want to know the kid's name, family situation, hopes and dreams, and what she likes to do—nail painting? Playing the ukulele? Snuggling with a stuffy? What does she think of the hospital food? Why is she ringing for the nurses, setting off alarms to bring the nurses back? Is she enjoying occupational therapy? When did she last have a bath or shower? How about the caregivers? Do they have caregiver fatigue? Who is supporting them? Those are things real doctors know about their patients. Many modern doctors don't know these things about their patients and actually care less. Those doctors will find the dollars do not come because the patients do not like that kind of care. They want something better.

Advice to doctors: Relate to your patients on their level and know who they are as persons. That knowledge will magnify your joy in practicing medicine. Furthermore, if you practice compassionate care, your practice will skyrocket. That's guaranteed.

My ironclad rule of medical economics is "Chase the dollars and they will never come. Take care of the patients and you will have so many dollars you won't know what to do with them."

Once, Stan Appel, Chair of Neurology at the time, accused me of "hogging all the patients." My answer was, "Just return their calls and you will have plenty of patients. It is that simple."

Yes, emphatic care requires the doctor to return patient calls, and emphatic care often requires repeated hospitalization, lots of nursing, and the involvement of specialists, occupational therapists, physical therapists, social workers, physician assistants, and dieticians whose time and efforts result in substantial expenditures.

In my view, emphatic medicine should be an integral part of scientific medicine and patchwork medicine. It can be. And sometimes is. Why not? Do you agree?

Summary: There are three main types of real medicine as discussed above.

1. Scientific Medicine

2. Patchwork Medicine—also known as technological medicine

3. Emphatic Medicine.

Next Up—Fake Medicine

Definition:

Fake medicine is anything that promises a health benefit but fails to deliver.

Fake medicine is all around you. Look around you. It is there.

Go to CVS or Walgreens and rummage through the long shelves of patent medicines for every conceivable real and imaginary illness. Note the small print on these patent medicines that usually says something like this: "The statements made have not been evaluated by the U.S Food and Drug Administration. This product is not intended to diagnose, cure, or prevent any illness. Testimonials are individual cases and do not guarantee that you will get the same results." How's that for a red flag! They use CYA (cover your ass) to get out of liability and to avoid accusations of false labeling and advertising.

Look at all the vitamins for sale. Vitamins are great and very profitable for those who make and sell them. For the rest of us, they are mainly a waste of time and money. Vitamins divide themselves into two groups: those that are water-soluble and those that are fat-soluble. Fat-soluble vitamins are A, D, E, and K. Because fat-soluble vitamins are stored in the human body's fat, it is easy to overdose on them. Serious illness and even death can result, and have resulted, from overdose of A or D. Major side effects occur with normal doses of E, including heart failure and bleeding. A study of 35,000 men showed a 17% increase in prostate cancer in those taking vitamin E compared to those taking a placebo. That study was in line with others that pretty much show if you try to prevent cancer with vitamins, you don't get helped and may get harmed. Men taking a multivitamin daily have a 36% greater chance of prostate cancer, according to a study by the University of Minnesota. Smokers (and asbestos workers) who took beta carotene as a supplement had a much greater chance of lung cancer than those who did not take beta carotene. Women who took one multivitamin a day have a 2.4% increased risk of early death compared to women who took no supplement. Vitamins K1 and K2 are probably safe, but K3 can produce liver damage in adults and brain damage in children.

Overdosing with water-soluble vitamins is hard to do because the human body has a great ability to piss out water-soluble vitamins. That's a good thing and the current estimate is that Americans piss out $63 million worth of these EACH DAY. Good thing! Otherwise, there would be lots of vitamin toxicity. But even overdose of some water-soluble vitamins can cause trouble. High doses of B6 (pyridoxal 5'phosphate) cause severe sensory neuropathy. B6 neuropathy has been reported with daily doses as low as 500 mg. It is ironic that in an effort to improve health, a person can damage nerves.

"Based on existing evidence, there is little justification for the general and widespread use of dietary supplements." Reference: Archives of Internal Medicine, 10/10/2011.

Take a look at the following health claims and judge for yourself. Compare your judgment with mine or that of the Federal Trade Commission (FTC):

Kellogg claimed that a breakfast of Frosted Mini-Wheats is "clinically shown to improve kids (sic) attentiveness by nearly 20%"

Your judgement, please.

FTC: The Company dropped the claim after the Federal Trade Commission filed suit.

General Mills said that by eating Cheerios, "you can lower your cholesterol 4% in 6 weeks."

Your judgment, please.

My judgment: Pure bunk

Kellogg offered Rice Krispies cereal, "now supports your child's immunity."

Your judgment:

My judgment: Pure bunk.

Nestle said the *Boost Kid Essentials* drink contains "probiotics clinically shown to help strengthen the immune system."

Your judgment:

FTC: Claim dropped after Federal Trade Commission suit.

General Foods promoted Postum as not just a beverage but as a cure for coffee drinking diseases. The moral fiber of coffee drinkers was seriously questioned until 1951, when, by agreement with the Federal Trade Commission, the company altered its advertisements so that they would not imply as they did that coffee "brews divorces, business failures, factory accidents, juvenile delinquency, traffic accidents, fire or home foreclosures."

POM Wonderful! (September 2010) Pomegranate juice was said "proven to fight for cardiovascular, prostate and erectile health" and leads to a "30% decrease in arterial plaque."

Your judgment:

FTC filed suit. Company lawyers say claims are scientifically validated. My prediction in 2010 was that the FTC would win after a long and costly legal battle. The Resnicks (Lynda and Stewart) who own POM are billionaires. Sometimes, the amount of money thrown on the scales of justice can influence the decisions, but most times, money merely delays what must happen eventually. There is no way that POM could, in my opinion, do all the things promised. Therefore, I conclude POM is a fake medicine because it promises what it can't deliver.

Result: The Federal Administrative Law Judge concluded that "POM Wonderful LLC and sister corporation Roll International and the principals Stewart Resnick, Lynda Resnick, and Mathew Tupper violated federal law by making deceptive disease prevention and treatment claims." The appeal court reached the same conclusion. On May 2, 2016 (note six years have gone by. The mills of justice grind exceedingly slow.), the United States Supreme Court refused to review the verdict—a final big blow to Stewart and Lynda. Evidently, the Supreme Court didn't think POM Wonderful! was wonderful enough. Further trouble for POM: On December 7, 2024, a class action against POM was certified. POM is being sued on the allegation that the product has perfluoro and polyfluoro chemicals, the so-called "forever chemicals," which seriously damage health.

Geritol is another example of health huckstering that reached tremendous proportions. Advertising became more powerful as technology allowed ways of reaching the masses, who are easily gulled. Geritol sponsored TV programs that catered largely to the older viewers: The Lawrence Welk Show, The Arthur Godfrey Show, What's My Line?, Ted Mack's Original Amateur Hour. Geritol was involved in the quiz show scandal as the sponsor of Twenty-One.

Pharmaceuticals, Inc., the distributor of Geritol, is reported to have spent $3 million a year in pre-1960 dollars advertising the preparation. As usual, the advertisers thought a lot more of the product than the majority of the medical profession and the FDA.

Ah! Geritol! The very name suggests it is good for the geriatric population. Aged and infirm persons provided a lucrative market for this product, which originally contained choline, methionine, and 12% alcohol. The alcohol was listed as a preservative, and no doubt it made some people feel better.

Geritol—What was it good for? Do you remember?

Tired blood!

Geritol's tired blood advertising included such claims as: If you feel run down because of TIRED BLOOD, FEEL STRONGER FAST within 7 days or money back....

> ...Take Geritol, the high potency tonic that begins to strengthen iron-poor, Tired Blood in just 24 hours.

> ....In a relatively short time, you can have what in a true sense amounts to a veritable blood transfusion....

> After an illness such as a cold, flu, sore throat or virus, you may suffer from Tired Blood. At such a time, GERITOL can help you regain your strength. It is one of the finest scientific blood-iron tonics yet created...

Take-home message:

There is a $23 billion per year industry out there trying to sell you supplements and minerals and stuff that are, for the most part, worthless junk that will not help you and may hurt you.

<u>Get your vitamins and minerals from real food and not from supplements.</u>

Fruits and vegetables are especially good for you, but supplements are not.

The Great Snake Oil Medicine Show

Picture this: It's 1880. You live in a small hick town in the southwest. There is no TV, no radio, no computer, no iPhone, no newspaper, and usually nothing happens, so you are bored stiff. Then, one bright sunny day, a medicine show arrives and sets up shop on Main Street with a clown who juggles and a barker dressed in a black suit with a top hat. He is addressed as Doctor, and no one thinks of questioning his credentials. After some entertainment, the real purpose of the medicine show begins. The Doctor touts the snake oil discovered by his learning its secrets from Walpi, Arizona Hopi Indian shamans. He shouts that this snake oil is a cure for anything that ails you, including all male troubles and all female troubles. There are even two men in the audience entourage who speak very highly of the snake oil. You haven't seen these guys before, but they look healthy. One says he lost his hearing and eyesight, and no doctor could help him, but within two weeks of taking snake oil, he was cured and has fully recovered his hearing and sight. The other guy says he had crippling arthritis with unbearable pain, all of which disappeared with this miracle treatment. He does a jig and shows hands that are arthritis free. Lots of bottles of snake oil are sold, and the doctor, the clown, the two shills, and the rest of the traveling medicine show move on to another town to dupe other rubes.

Yes, from that humble beginning, with the assistance of massive newspaper advertising and public relations and multiple testimonials from real and unreal patients, and the endorsements from prominent members of Congress, snake oil became the most resorted-to patent medical treatment in America. As usual, though, the truth surfaced and won out. In 1917, the United States government tested snake oil at Clark Stanley's snake oil factory in Massachusetts. The product contained mineral oil, capsaicin, and turpentine, but no snake oil. The government concluded that this product was fake snake oil and fined Clark $20 for mislabeling his patent medicine. The public was outraged for being duped, and snake oil disappeared only to be replaced by another patent medicine called Peruna.

Peruna was the invention of Samuel Hartmann, a physician, surgeon, and multimillionaire quack. He redefined catarrh as the cause of all disease. Catarrh was once a kind of valid diagnosis to describe congestion of the throat that we might now call posterior nasal drip from a common cold or post-nasal mucus from air pollution. Hartmann declared that catarrh was not only that but also the cause of all diseases. Pneumonia was catarrh of the lungs, tuberculosis was a form of catarrh, appendicitis ditto, mumps ditto, yellow fever ditto, Bright's disease (kidney failure) ditto, and so forth. The cure of catarrh was Peruna, a patent medicine endorsed by 50 members of Congress and many entertainers. At the peak, Hartmann earned over $100,000 a day (yes, a day! Think of what that would be in today's dollars!) from Peruna sales, and over half the households in America had Peruna on board. No kidding.

The end came after a series of articles written by Samuel Adams entitled *The Great American Fraud* were published in Collier's magazine. Peruna was exposed as containing 28% alcohol. In an interview, Hartmann himself admitted to Adams that Peruna was of no medical value unless someone believed in it, and then the placebo effect would make Peruna look partially effective. Aye, there's the rub. Patent medicine often has and has had a placebo effect. Hartmann died January 30, 1918, at his own hotel, the Hartmann Hotel. Legend has it he refused Peruna as a treatment for his pneumonia.

Is that the end of it? No way. A modern replacement will always surface to dupe the public. The latest appears to be Top Gun USA.

According to the information on the internet:

"Top Gun is a revolutionary brain supplement formulated to give you ultimate brain power. Known in Scientific Terms as a "NOOTROPIC" or "GENIUS PILL," Top Gun improves mental functions such as cognition, memory, intelligence, motivation, attention, concentration, and therefore, **happiness** and **success**. You will be limitless!

It goes on:

"Top Gun is so effective that you will have lightning-fast thinking under any circumstances, including a genius-level boost when you are tired, have brain fog, or even after a heavy night of drinking. Don't let the demands of a job, school, or social life slow you down. Top Gun maximizes your concentration with ultimate efficiency so that you have more time for the things you and your brain would rather be doing!"

And on and on it goes, explaining the benefits to working memory, information processing, nerve growth in the brain, increased blood flow and oxygen to the brain, and more.

I have waded through pages and pages of this hype and read two of the supporting testimonials: one by John D. of Fort Lauderdale, who no longer crams for exams and who believes, "This stuff is almost a miracle!" and one by Jane M. from Bakersfield, who says she is no longer "ditzy," feels like a rocket scientist, and everyone likes and trusts her now.

More: Top Gun is the #1 choice for cognition enhancement. Premium Brain Supplement. It will help you "Blow Away the Competition at Job Interviews, Work or School"

The advertisement also has two brain scans—one before and one after Top Gun. Both scans are fake. The "after" scan shows lights in ten brain regions, all of which were add-ons to the picture to make it look like Top Gun lit up the brain like a Christmas decoration.

Blow Away the Competition at Job Interviews, Work or School

Reduce Stress and Increase Your Happiness and Success Quotients

Turbo-Charge
Key Aspects of Brain Power

Top Gun clinically scientifically stimulates four areas of brain power, focus, attention, memory and overall brain health. That means working results everywhere you go.

▶

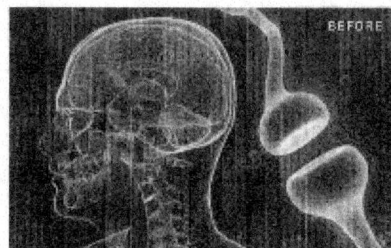
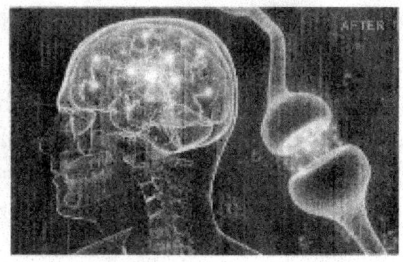

Attention and Focus   Unlock Long-Term Memory

Last page but one says "Warning: Due to extremely high media demand, there is a limited supply of Top Gun as of 6th of December 2024. HURRY!"

On the last page, in small print, there appears the usual statement that the product has not been approved by the Food and Drug Administration. And guess what? It also says the product is not intended to diagnose, cure, or prevent any disease. And it adds—The testimonials on this website are individual cases and do not guarantee that you will get the same results. There is more CYA (cover your ass), but I will spare you, dear reader. You get the point. But, if you are about to order some Top Gun, STOP! First, deal with me. There is a bridge in Brooklyn I want to sell to you.

On and on, the fakes continue unabated. Carter's Little Liver Pills are still out there, except the Federal Trade Commission made them take the liver away from the title, so now it's just Carter's Little Pills. Lydia Pinkham's herbal is still available for female troubles. Lydia seemed to reply to letters from fans for a very long time. The product lost some fans when Ladies Home Journal showed a picture of Lydia's tombstone proving the reply letters were not from Lydia.

For exercise, take a look at Gwyneth Paltrow's website (gwynethpaltrow.com) and draw your own conclusions about GOOP.

Sometimes the past is a prologue that we can learn from and hope not to make the same mistakes.

Here's an example of mainstream medicine that got it wrong and touted a treatment that turned out to be fake. Remember the definition of fake medicine? Fake medicine promises a health benefit but fails to deliver. A startling example is frontal lobotomy.

Lobotomy (Cutting the Frontal Lobe of the Brain)—An International Medical Fad

Rosemarie Kennedy, sister of JFK, had a difficult birth. Because a physician was not immediately available at the labor, Rose's mother was advised by a nurse to hold her legs closed until the doctor arrived. The child remained in the birth canal for about two hours, during which she probably suffered brain damage due to low brain oxygen. Result: Rosemarie was retarded. Despite special education, she, at age 9-10, was reading at a fourth-grade level, but was actually happy and reasonably functional in the activities of daily life. At about age 22, she became "irritable and difficult," and her father, without telling the mother, arranged for Rosemarie to have a frontal lobotomy. The official diagnosis at the time was depression. The real reason for Joseph Kennedy's concern is not known. People speculate he was concerned about possible promiscuity, but there was no evidence that Rosemarie was wired that way.

The 1941 operation was done by neurosurgeon James W. Watts with the assistance of neurologist Walter Freeman. They gave a tranquillizer to relax Rose, made two holes in her skull, and asked her to recite The Lord's Prayer as they cut the prefrontal lobe of her brain with a spatula. When Rose became incoherent, they stopped cutting.

Result: The operation caused immense harm. Rose's I.Q. declined to that of a two-year-old. She couldn't walk, spoke gibberish, and was incontinent of urine and stool. The sparkle of her personality was gone forever. She had become apathetic and lethargic. Loss of personality and personal sparkle was and is the most common side effect of the operation.

Rose eventually recovered a little, but not enough. She remained incapacitated for the rest of her life and spent the next 63 years at various institutions, but mainly at Saint Colletta, in Jefferson, Wisconsin. (Saint Colletta is the patron of sick children.)

Tennessee Williams' older sister, Rose, same story: after lobotomy, incapacitated for life. In fact, the same story for the most part for the 40,000 people operated on in the United States and the 17,000 in England, and the 9,300 in Scandinavia.

Many gay men had the procedure to change their sexual orientation and make them "morally sane." No detailed follow-up studies were done on them or anyone. No placebo group used for comparison. Therefore, this was work unscientific in the extreme. Almost any mental illness was considered O.K. for this treatment, including childhood misbehaviors (popular in Japan even at age two), hysteria, chronic pain (Eva Peron was operated for pain three months before her death), depression, panic attacks, and schizophrenia. Lobotomy was even used as a way to prevent subsequent mental illness, a sort of prophylactic. Walter Freeman, who was famous for doing 25 mass production operations a day, said we have "to nip mental illness in the bud." He did the operation on anyone who he thought might develop a mental illness. No question Freeman got carried away, cultivating the media and doing over 3,000 lobotomies until his surgical privileges were removed. He continued to claim the operation was a tremendous success despite the massive evidence to the contrary. You would think the very poor result with Rosemarie Kennedy and many others would have dampened public enthusiasm for lobotomy, but it didn't.

It would be instructive to know why and how this dangerous fad continued so long and was so widely practiced. We really don't know, nor can we fully explain this troubling story of how mainstream medicine got it so wrong for so long. I admit I don't understand it. But here are some ideas to consider:

The past is a different country. They do things differently there. It was an era when there were no effective treatments for mental illnesses. Physicians and families were at their wits' end. The asylums were filled with the insane who received only custodial care, much of which was very poor indeed. The lobotomy promised a lot (rah rah for that) but delivered little in the way of benefits and lots in the way of fever, brain hemorrhage, bowel and bladder incontinence, apathy, akinesia, lethargy, and death. Yes, death. Surgical mortality was 5%. I guess you could make the case that lobotomy made total care easier, as the individual's personality was erased and was no longer there to complain or fight back. Killing the patients also made total care easier and less expensive. Ken Kesey (Jack Nicholson's character), after a lobotomy in the film *One Flew Over the Cuckoo's Nest*, was no longer a troublemaker for Nurse Ratched or anyone else. Ken was cured of his personality and his vitality, and he was now of no more use to himself or others.

Equally puzzling was the award of the Nobel Prize in Medicine to Egas Moniz in 1949. I always thought the prize went to Moniz for his invention of cerebral arteriography with injection of sodium iodide. But I was wrong. The official citation says it was for the surgical treatment of psychiatric disease. Thorstein Wiesel called this prize "an astounding (error) of judgment ... a terrible mistake." Other notable doctors called it "the worst Nobel ever." Moniz shared the prize with Walter Hess, who demonstrated that he could make a cat fall asleep by stimulating certain sections of the hypothalamus. I don't think that is such a great achievement. My cats are very good at falling asleep on their own without any special help from anyone.

Lesson: Maintain a healthy skepticism about all health claims. Do not over-exercise the believing centers of your brain. Ask questions. Go with the facts and not with the hype. Be an informed health skeptic.

Chiropractic—Another Example of Health Hucksters

You probably already know what I was about to write about this form of fake medicine. But instead of writing what I think, I will let others speak for me:

"…the teachers, research workers and practitioners of medicine reject the so-called principle on which chiropractic is based and correctly and bluntly label it a fraud and hoax on the human race…" -Milton Helpern, M.D., Chief Medical Examiner of the City of New York

"The theory which underlies chiropractic is false… Biology is probably the most complex and difficult of sciences and human biology its most important branch. To reduce to one primary mechanical concept is single-minded and dangerous." -Extracts from a statement by the Faculty of Medicine of McGill University to the Commission on Chiropractic, Quebec.

"Chiropractic theory and practice are not based upon the body of basic knowledge related to health, disease and health care that has been widely accepted by the scientific community Moreover, irrespective of its theory, the scope and quality of chiropractic education do not prepare the practitioner to make an adequate diagnosis and provide appropriate treatments." -Report, U.S. Department of Health, Education and Welfare, 1968.

"Chiropractic theory claims that human disease is ultimately caused by pressure on spinal nerves. Chiropractors have treated diseases ranging from the common cold to meningitis and cancer by manipulation of the spine. Therefore, it is recommended that chiropractic services not be covered by the Medicare program. -Ralph Lee Smith in his book entitled *at your own risk, the case against CHIRO-PRACTIC*, 1969, Pocket Books, New York.

Lesson: Forget spinal adjustments. Beyond placebo effects, they don't work. In some cases, they are dangerous and have led to significant harm or delay in correct treatment or both.

Spas

Some spas are great, and some are not so great. My own experience has been good. Whenever I stay at a hotel, I seek out the spa. While traveling 91 days around the world on the Queen Elizabeth 2, I hardly ever missed a daily trip to the spa. There, I enjoyed the whirlpool, the steam room, the sauna, as well as the company of many other passengers who became my friends. At Hot Springs National Park, I enjoyed the mud bath followed by the cold bath and massage.

When I was a visiting professor in Montpellier, France, I learned how medical care can be conditioned by culture. If a man came to the clinic saying he felt sad and was crying often and had suicidal thoughts every 27 seconds, we, in the United States, would probably conclude that the patient needed hospitalization and mood-elevating drugs and maybe even electroshock treatment. Not so in France. In France, the diagnosis was "Crise de Fois"—liver crisis. Since this patient's crise de fois is serious, the indicated treatment was a two-week vacation at a spa in Biarritz for thalassotherapy (sea water treatments) at government expense. And believe it or not, the patient usually returned healthy and free of what we would have called major depression.

It has not been shown that the mineral content of the waters has any particular benefit. In all probability, the benefit of the spa is simply a matter of rest and relaxation. A trip away from the office or away from home itself is often a trip away from worries, tensions, and frustrations associated with everyday life, a change of scenery—these in themselves are often instrumental in producing rest and relaxation, which are beneficial. As for me, I like a warm bath at home each night. It is a nice way to get relaxed for bed.

So, spa if you like, the way I do, without any special expectation of a health benefit. It is just a way to pass some time, and it definitely helps me adjust my physical and mental attitude. Do it if it pleases you, and don't do it if it doesn't.

America's most famous spa no longer exists. It was the spa at Battle Creek, Michigan, a kind of high-class hotel, state-of-the-art hospital, European Spa, and resort. Originally called the sanatorium (the place of rest for weary veterans), the name was changed to sanitarium by alteration of two letters, and later it was known simply as the San.

Over 300,000 patients seeking health passed through its exercise rooms and lecture hall and cold-water baths and salt water showers, and the basement bowel and rectal douches service, and so forth. Among the patients were some notables like Thomas Edison, President Taft, Amelia Earhart, Henry Ford, Mary Todd Lincoln, J.C. Penny, Montgomery Ward, Harvey Firestone, C.W. Post, James Buick, and the grape juice baron Edgar Welch. You can learn more about the Spa from the book *The Road to Wellville* by T.C. Boyle and the 1994 movie by the same title, where Anthony Hopkins plays the director of the spa, Doctor John Harvey Kellogg. By the way, the title *The Road to Wellville* is the title of a best-selling book by C.W. Post, the cereal king, wherein he outlines his ideas for health and happiness. C.W. Post's book didn't help him fully recover his own health. After nine months at the San, he was discharged as hopeless. On May 10, 1914, alone in his bedroom, he placed the muzzle of a rifle in his mouth and pulled the trigger with his toe. He was 59. He left $33 million, mainly to his daughter Marjorie. She died at age 86. Her 118-room Palm Beach palace, Mar-a-Lago, became the showcase possession of Donald J. Trump.

Doctor Kellogg's ideas on health were not far off in some matters. He believed in fresh air, exercise, and a good diet of mainly vegetables. He was down on corsets (they obstructed breathing), alcohol, tobacco, coffee, and tea. He was sure tobacco was a cause of lung cancer and wrote one of the earliest papers on the subject. According to him, coffee and tea made people nervous and nonproductive and depressed and weak, and tired all the time. That tired all the time led to a new diagnosis called neurasthenia, for which electric baths were prescribed. Smoking was forbidden at the San because it supposedly damaged the liver. Alcohol, coffee, and tea were never served at the San.

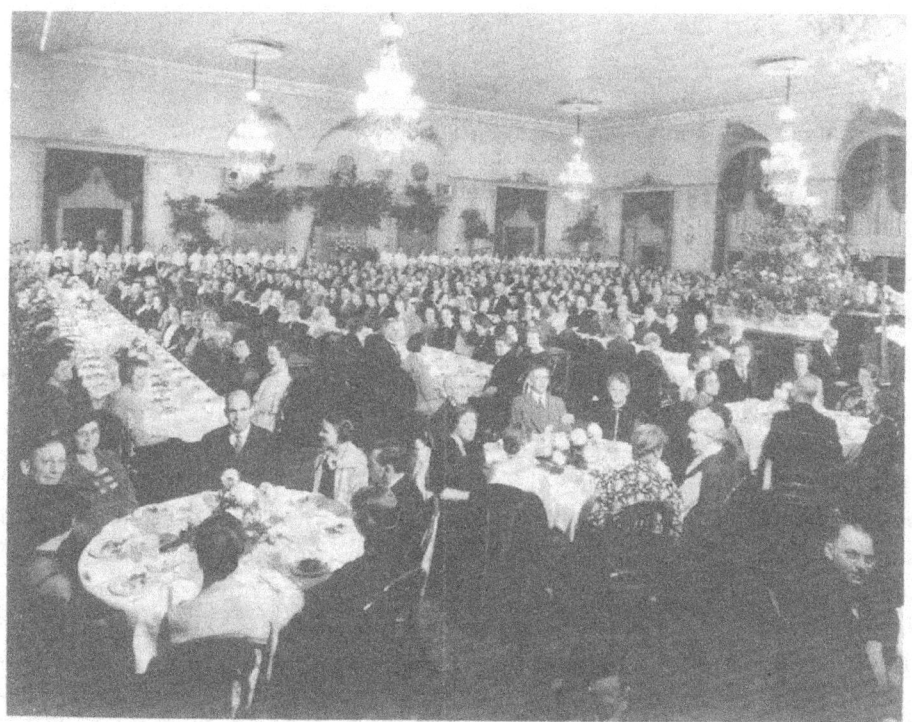

52. Early twentieth-century dining at the San was no spartan affair. *Courtesy, Historical Society of Battle Creek.*

Modern medicine considers coffee and tea in moderate amounts okay. Alcohol is considered a food, a sacrament, a poison, or a drug depending on the situation and particular use. You could argue pro and con for these things. Use your judgment.

On the other hand, some of Doctor Kellogg's ideas were way off. He was especially fond of enemas. He started every day with one for himself. Followed by yogurt by mouth and per rectum. Patients at the San had frequent enemas, whether they needed them or not. Usually, they got an enema five days a week and not on the weekends. I guess *toxic colon disease*, the major diagnosis at the San, took a holiday on the weekends. Even in modern times, X-ray therapy and chemo are not given on the weekends because everyone knows cancers don't grow on the weekends.

Kellogg abhorred constipation and blamed it as the source of "auto-intoxication," that is, the poisoning of the human body. In his own words, "Universal constipation is the most destructive blockage that has ever opposed human progress." As a surgeon, he performed over 20,000 operations, many of which were for the relief of a kink in the colon (known as "Lane's kink"), a disease he felt significantly impaired healthy digestion and resulted in many physical signs and symptoms. The usual definition of a kink is a sharp twist or curve. Will, the patient in the movie *The Road to Wellville,* gets his kink removed by Doctor Kellogg. Everyone has a kink in their colon, where stasis usually occurs; that's normal. But according to Doctor Kellogg, patient Will needed the kink removed by abdominal surgery. The kinked colon idea as a cause of disease is now passé, as is the idea of autointoxication from normal conditions of the intestines. Hydrotherapy, phototherapy, electrotherapy, and mechanotherapy (with a special machine that shakes you up) were among what we moderns might call questionable therapeutic tools.

Also, objectionable according to modern standards is the inhalation of Radon from the radioactive decay of Radium (atomic number 88). Nice historic pictures of a woman inhaling radon are in T.C. Boyle's book, *Part II* Therapeutics, pages 164-165. Doctor Kellogg called this his most efficacious cure for chlorosis (chlorosis also known as Green Disease, which we now know what Doctor Kellogg did not know, was a greenish facial complexion caused by iron deficiency anemia) and a host of other conditions, including erysipelas (skin infection), obesity, and ingrown toenails. The Curies had discovered radium and polonium and won the 1903 Nobel Prize in Physics. Doctor Kellogg picked right up on it, using this "healing" metal (radon is an alkali metal that is silver white) that Doctor Kellogg thought gave off rays and vibrations, which he called emanations. Radon (atomic number 86) is a noble gas. Therefore, it is inert, colorless, odorless, and tasteless. Inhaling it is carcinogenic because of the decay daughters, which emit alpha particles, beta particles, and gamma rays. The most common cause of lung cancer is smoking, but the second most common cause is radon exposure. Among non-smokers who get lung cancer, radon is the most common cause of lung cancer. The exposure is worldwide and most often occurs without people knowing they are exposed. When I was in France in 1981, large exposures were documented among people who lived in stone houses because the stones have small amounts of radium, which decays to radon, which then accumulated in poorly ventilated basements. The health consequences of inhaling radon at the Spa must have been significant, but no one knew how serious they were at the time, and there was no follow-up.

Furthermore, Doctor Kellogg was against sex in any manner, shape, or form. He recommended severe punishments for children who discovered masturbating. Though married for decades, he claimed he never consummated the marriage. He and his wife, Ella, had separate bedrooms and no natural children. Sex was among the "baser appetites." All married couples at the San were required to have separate bedrooms and were cautioned about how unhealthy sex was. Doctor Kellogg felt sex wasted vital body fluids, making you weak and causing premature death. He considered an erect penis the "flag pole of death." About Kellogg's disdain for sex in any form, modern medicine has lots to say, mainly by way of disagreement.

The San's policy against sex is difficult to understand. It seems wrong from the start. Without sex, the human race is doomed to extinction. Right? Hence, sex seems natural and, in fact, it is natural for all the other animals on this planet. Why would human animals be any different?

What's your view: Is sex good or not? Was the San right by coming out dead set against sex, condemning sex in any manner or form?

The Modern View

You don't need a doctor to tell you that regular sex relieves stress, improves sleep, and increases intimacy with your partner. Some evidence says sex improves immunity and makes you look better. In fact, a Scottish study showed couples with a healthy sex life may look up to seven years younger than those with a ho-hum bedroom ritual. Sex probably increases longevity—at least that is what my 94-year-old mother-in-law believed. She thought the effect is due to "tricking your body into thinking you are reproducing." British studies agree with her by showing that men who have sex once a week live ten years longer on average than those who have sex once a month. A Duke University study showed that women who are happy with their sex life live seven to eight years longer than those who are unhappy with their sex life. Science tells us that sex releases endorphins, the body's natural painkillers, which is why sex brings temporary relief from back pain, migraines, and other body aches. Most studies show that people who have sex often have fewer heart attacks and strokes. This may be a chicken or egg effect, for we don't know what comes first. Does sex prevent vascular disease, or is it rather a fact that those people who don't have vascular disease are more likely to have sex, or is it both those two things: healthy people have more sex, and more sex makes for more health? Some evidence indicates that sex prevents cancer. This is particularly true of prostate cancer. Emptying the tank is probably good for the prostate. And last but not least, sex is FUN, and you may even get a baby out of it. And if you don't get a baby—so what!

Why did I do this exposition on sex at the San?

Answer: I wanted to show that the San, a world-famous health resort run by a world-famous doctor and visited by many people, most of whom were rich and many of whom were world famous, did in fact issue medical advice about sex that was completely wrong.

Besides doing a terrible job on normal sex, the San did a terrible job on the patients who had Green Disease. This was a hypochromic anemia that was due to iron deficiency. The usual victim was a woman who had lost blood via her monthly. These ladies were so pale they looked like a victim of Bram Stoker's monsters, sucked dry of blood. Because of the anemia, these women had pale faces that sometimes looked slightly green, hence the name Green Disease. Vegetarian diet is a no-no for such patients because vegetables have little iron. What the ladies needed was iron or some food like red meat, which has lots of iron. This information was not known at the time, and consequently, Green Disease caused lots of weakness, fatigue, apathy, and even death. Miss Muntz in the movie *The Road to Wellville* dies of her Green Disease anemia. Meat was sometimes on the menu at the San, but anyone ordering it was frowned upon. Those with Green Disease had to remain on a vegetarian diet, which was for them the kiss of death.

Why all this bad medicine at the San? Who knows? And why did all those doctors on the staff (up to 30) and all those nurses go along with the stupid policies of the San? Why did the patients tolerate a 15-gallon enema in the mornings? Why did they risk their lives taking electric shock therapy even after some of the technicians died of electrocution? These are very big questions, and there are some very big lessons here:

1. Watch out. Just because a physician, spa, or hospital has a good reputation does not necessarily mean they will be right for your particular health needs.

2. A doctor's reputation can be a fluke merely based on his/her association with a well-known university or hospital. I have personally witnessed some major errors made by the chairmen of the departments of neurology. One told a patient they had amyotrophic lateral sclerosis and would probably die in three years. The diagnosis was wrong. Thirty years later, that patient is still going strong. Another chairman was treating a patient for Lupus when the correct diagnosis was Ehrlichiosis, an infection by an intracellular bacterium spread by tick bite and treatable with antibiotics and not corticosteroids. A chairman diagnosed a patient as having progressive familial paralysis when there was no family history of the same, and subsequent removal of a herniated cervical disc cured the problem. A patient of mine had been to the Mayo Clinic, where she was thought to have cancer somewhere because she was so weak. They did lots of tests, including radiographic examination of the stomach and small intestine, barium enema, gall bladder studies, intravenous pyelogram to look at the kidney and ureters, and bladder, and finally an exploratory laparotomy—all of which turned out negative for cancer. The post-operative course was "rocky," and my patient signed out against medical advice. When she arrived in my clinic in a wheelchair, she did look like she was at death's door. But a review of the Mayo records showed the electrolyte abnormalities of adrenal insufficiency. And indeed, her blood cortisol was zero. She rose from the dead with a proper replacement of corticosteroid, two pills a day. Her husband owned an oil pipe company in Houston and became a major supporter of my research.

How do I explain such mistakes? Easy. We all make mistakes—me too. But also, a chairman may not be a great clinician. He/she may instead be a great administrator or great business person. They may have gotten where they are because of their political acumen, or their research reputation, or because they were simply lucky, or were good brown nosers. Csaba Szabo, a professor at the University of Fribourg, has an interesting cartoon in his new book *Unreliable*: The recruitment committee is looking at three candidates for a job. One is a plagiarist, one is a cheat, and the third is a sexual harasser, and they decide to go with the one with the most grant money. But it's not a joke. --- I have seen this kind of thing.

In part two, which is about to begin, we will relive some excellent examples of why you need to be alert and cautious about your health care decisions. Do your best to make sure the doctor and the proposed tests and treatments are right for you. Your life depends on it.

Faith Healing

Forget it. You will be disappointed. Beyond a placebo effect, faith does not work. Stick to science. Religion often gets it wrong. The story I can't resist telling is about the Millerites. They picked several dates for the Second Coming of Christ, finally settling on October 22, 1844. Their faith was confirmed by various "signs" such as earthquakes, shooting stars, and a comet in the winter sky over North America in March 1843. As the big day approached, believers (there were over 50,000 of them) gave away their homes, quit their jobs, and waited on hilltops to be swept into paradise. When the Savior didn't show, many were crushed. But I would bet they still all voted straight Republican.

Historians refer to the event as "The Great Disappointment." Millerites were just one of many. Backed by religious certainty, end-of-world predictions started with Jewish Essenes (70 A.D.) and run through several hundred up to Jeane Dixon (2020). Jeane had previously predicted February 4, 1962, but as usual, nothing happened. Martin Luther came in on 1600, but Jesus again failed to show even for him. Pope Sylvester II came in on January 1, 1000, part of the millennial craze. Then there was a revision to 1033 on the idea that the world would end 1,000 years after Jesus died. Pope Innocent III came in in 1284 on the theory that the world would end 666 years after the establishment of Islam. Again, the Savior didn't show even for Popes, his representatives on Earth.

Religious maniacs bring multitudes of believers together as few demagogues can, and with the force of conviction the latter can't inspire. So what? What does all of this prove? All this proves that craziness is a common human failing. The herd wants to believe and will believe what they want to believe. Never over-exercise the believing sections of your brain. Stay objective and stick to the facts. Practice the art of clear and logical thinking. If you don't know what that art entails, read Rolf Dobelli's book *The Art of Thinking Clearly*.

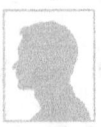

PART TWO
MODERN MEDICAL ENCOUNTERS

PART TWO—MODERN MEDICAL ENCOUNTERS

◆ ◆ ◆

"Life is what happens when you are not watching TV."

— Bernard Patten

My modern medical life experience divides itself into two sections:

Section A: Experience as a doctor

Section B: Experience as a patient

First, Section A—The Experience as a Doctor

"Doctors are great—as long as you don't need them."

— Doctor Edward E. Rosenbaum's Grandmother

My medical career started in June 1966 when I graduated from the College of Physicians and Surgeons of Columbia University (P&S). After that, many highly regarded institutions trusted me for decades. I want you to trust me, too, and I want you to believe what I am about to tell you is true, and that is why I will summarize (briefly) my qualifications as a practitioner.

My internship was straight medicine at the great white erection on the east side of Manhattan, the New York Hospital—Cornell Medical Center. After that, I returned to Columbia as an assistant resident neurologist and then Chief Resident Neurologist at the Neurological Institute of New York. The next year, I was the Raisbeck Memory Fellow of the New York Academy of Medicine and founded and directed the memory clinic at Columbia. At age 30, I had to do my draft obligated service as assistant chief of medical neurology at the National Institutes of Health. There, I took care of patients admitted to the clinical center and did the neurological consultations for the center and for National Naval Medical Center, and occasionally for Walter Reed Hospital. It was also part of my duty to care for the neurological needs of the people in the United States Senate and the House of Representatives.

At NIH, I had my own laboratory and my own technician (Katherine Oliver) and did research on neuromuscular transmission and the mechanisms of action of nerve gases. We published papers in major medical journals and received many awards from medical societies and from foundations.

After demobilization, in 1973, I joined the faculty of the Baylor College of Medicine as the Chief of Nerve and Muscle Diseases and Vice Chair of the Department of Neurology. For decades, I had the largest and most varied neurological practice in the world at Methodist Hospital, Saint Luke's Hospital, and Texas Children's Hospital. I helped train hundreds of medical students, many residents, and 123 fellows.

I gave over 500 lectures to various national and international medical groups and, for 22 years, did oral examinations for the American Board of Psychiatry and Neurology to determine who was qualified to practice neurology as a specialist. I was a visiting professor at the Cleveland Clinic, Henry Ford Hospital, Beaumont Army Hospital, Charcot Clinic in Paris, Louisiana State University, Charity Hospital, Tulane Medical School, Karolinska University Hospital, Karolinska Institute, Sweden, the Major Social Security Hospital, Lisbon, and the University of Montpellier in southern France, and so forth.

The practice was wonderful, and I loved taking care of people. My specialty was the very sick who had complicated medical problems. Thank God I had an army of nurses, residents, and fellows who helped take care of patients.

All was hunky-dory until about 1990, when the trouble started.

Until about 1990, as I view it, insurance was a legitimate business. The way it worked was simple. The insurance company had a smart group of accountants and actuaries who were able to estimate with great accuracy the yearly risks of various conditions in a given group of people in a certain location. They then predicted how much the company would have to pay out in benefits and added a small amount to that number (say, 20%) for profits. That mathematical work determined how much the company would need from premiums to pay for the few policyholders who got sick. That is the basic principle of indemnification as I understand it. You spread individual risk among many people who each pay a small premium for protection if they get sick.

The system worked well, and I swear to you in the golden age of medicine, there was no real concern about money and no real problem collecting what was due from the health insurance companies. I would send in my bill, and the insurance would send me a check pretty quickly without any question or dispute.

In or about 1990, things seemed to change. I wish I had kept careful records of what happened, but I didn't because I was too busy taking care of patients. So, what you are about to read is basically from my memory, which is pretty good, but not perfect. My memory research warns me to beware of what I write and be objective. Memories of our past can be largely a self-serving construct with a few facts thrown in.

An insurance company demanded in a letter, "Doctor, explain in exact detail what you did for this patient."

I had never received a letter like that, and I was puzzled because the company had already received a detailed four-page single-spaced discharge summary of how I had saved the patient's life. Despite the information they already had, they were asking me to further justify my bill. Naughty me! I turned their letter on its side and scribbled in bright blue ink: "I worried. Pay up."

Cora, my secretary, sent their letter back to them with my comment. One week later, the check came for the full amount billed. That was nice, but after that auspicious beginning, lots of trouble and stormy weather followed.

The companies (some of them, not all) seemed to be operating under a new system designed to delay payment, and later to deny payment and still later to defend nonpayment in court. The insurance business was becoming a scam in which what was promised was not delivered. WellCare was an offender, and so was Cigna. But the worst of them was, in my opinion, Blue Cross and Blue Shield. Humana, on the other hand, was good.

It took a while, but eventually I caught on. My attitude changed. I concluded the companies were now money hungry and had invented a host of little tricks to lower payment or prevent payment. These tricks were invented, I believe, to increase profits because what is not paid out to policyholders as a benefit becomes money for stockholder dividends and for CEOs' (Chief Executive Officers) salaries. Many CEOs I discovered had gigantic salaries, much more than mine, but the salary was not their major take-home compensation. No way! Stock options and other advanced tax gimmicks gave them millions. My guess is that CEO Brian Thomson, for instance, took (he was killed in New York City with bullets labelled delay, deny, defend) home more money each year than any doctor, including any cardiovascular surgeon. That is wrong, dead wrong. That is wrong because the money the company got should have gone to the policyholders to pay for the medical bills that were becoming a gigantic problem for many households. In a practical sense, people were insured until they got sick, and then they had to work to collect what they were entitled to get paid.

Although I was sympathetic to my patients' plight, in many cases, I was unable to help. The policy terms had been carefully written by the insurance companies to favor the companies over the policyholders. The result was that what the patients thought was covered was either not covered or not covered in full because of the long list of exclusions, exceptions, loopholes, chintziness, and idiosyncratic interpretations of definitions.

Conditions were also a problem. Conditions are different from exclusions. If the policy says you must notify the plan of an emergency before you enter the hospital for your heart attack—that is a condition of coverage—and if you didn't notify the plan for whatever reason, then the admission is not covered. Some patients are too sick or too stupid, or too frightened, to do the prenotification. Hence, denial of coverage.

Consequent to the denials, patients spend lots of time on the phone and lots of time writing letters, lots of time fighting the red tape and the bullshit, and some time (usually very brief) appearing at appeals to try to collect what should have been paid. The rigamarole is what I consider a major hidden cost of insurance. Those of you who have had this experience know exactly what I am talking about, and those of you who have not had this experience (yet) will have it sometime in the future.

Improper denials of coverage are a fact of life in modern medicine.

Oh, you children of the future, make up your mind that you will spend a fair amount of time keeping your insurance company from keeping your money.

In most cases, I was of little help in defending patients from insurance abuse until I made a eureka discovery. There were denials based on the idea that the test I ordered or the surgery I did, or the medicine I prescribed was not medically necessary.

Ho ho ho.

Now I knew I had them. The companies could not know anywhere near what I knew about medicine, and they were behind the power curve because they had not done a history, a physical examination, and a neurological examination. I had. They were significantly behind the power curve because they didn't know boo or beans about the disease the patient had or the complications thereof.

The fundamental problem is the hunger for money. Health plans manage care whether you like it or not. They manage care by managing costs. They manage costs by limiting their payments for services, procedures, treatments, and medicines. The most common trick is to claim that XXXXX is not medically necessary. The problem is that the plan has a financial interest in deciding that things are not necessary, and in some recent contracts, I have seen specific language that affirms that the plan, and only the plan, decides what is and what is not necessary. In other words, the plan is in control, and your doctor is not in control. What counts is what the plan thinks. Sad, sad, and very sad. This is not good for the doctor, and it is not good for you, the patient.

I think that money hunger also led to the misguided perspective that health care is in a binary world in which interventions are either effective or not effective, appropriate or inappropriate. The truth is there are lots of gray zones in which the care is neither clearly justified nor not clearly justified—zones whose benefits are unknown or uncertain and whose value may depend on the patient's preference and the available alternatives. Gray zones are the rule when we deal with previously unrecognized diseases, new treatments, or new techniques.

What I Did to Try to Abate the Situation

Acting on behalf of my patients and with their full permission, I argued their case in court. Usually, the issue went before an administrative law judge. The two opposition lawyers were usually poorly prepared and knew little. Some of them didn't even feel like defending the companies they were working for. I could tell by body language and facial expressions that their hearts were not in it. Deep down in their deep hearts' cores, I believe they thought the company was wrong. Yes, many of the attorneys in the interest of justice would slough the case or admit a mistake has been made and move that the judge order payment. Some did not actually admit a mistake, but when the judge asked for their statements in defense, they simply said that they had nothing to say! In one case, the judge asked again: "You have nothing to say? What kind of defense is that?" To which question, both opposing lawyers said in unison: "Your honor, we have nothing to say."

I won all cases—about 48 cases. In general, the judges saw right through the arguments of the companies or their non-arguments. The usual judicial statement went like this: "The attending physician is in a much better position to decide what is medically necessary than the insurance company."

Example: Insurance denied payment for magnetic scan (MRI) of the brain in a patient who had suspected multiple sclerosis. They said the use of MRI was "unapproved" and "medically unnecessary." That was stupid. MRI was unapproved by their self-serving attitude. But MRI was definitely approved by the majority of neurologists as a reasonable clinical tool.

The magnetic scan confirmed the clinically suspected diagnosis and showed very severe disease throughout the brain. The severity indicated that powerful treatments were needed to bring the disease under control. Following a Harvard protocol for severe multiple sclerosis, I administered Cytoxan. The spinal fluid markers of multiple sclerosis, oligoclonal bands, and intra-blood-brain barrier immune globulin G production disappeared, and so did the clinical signs and symptoms of the disease. Thirty years later, I met the patient at the Greek Festival in Clear Lake, Texas. She had been bussed in with her retirement home friends. She was disease-free and fully functional and had been normal without any further treatment. Wow! If I had severe multiple sclerosis, that would be the treatment I would consider, but only after I looked at my MRI.

Result: The judge thought the MRI in my patient's case was fully justified: "The doctor, not a company, should be making the decisions about what is or what is not needed." And of course, the insurance company lost and had to pay $800 for the MRI plus interest. Scans were cheaper in the old days, or money was more valuable, or both.

In one trial, I did lose the case initially. It was against Blue Cross and Blue Shield (BCBS), which claimed I had over-coded outpatient visits. My average code was 2.8, with 3 being the usual code for the usual average visit. The codes run from 1 to 5, and in my view, if anything, I had undercoded. The two lawyers opposed to me put a young neurologist on the stand as their witness. Strangely, he said he had examined the clinical records very carefully and had concluded that I was correct. He coded the visits a big fat 4! His testimony was that I had undercoded and was due a refund and additional payments.

Hot dog! Now, silly me, I thought I had to win about claw back because not only did I have the facts on my side and the law on my side, and the patients on my side, I also had their expert witness on my side.

The Blue Cross and Blue Shield lawyers were unhappy and told the judge that the testimony of the young neurologist should be disregarded because, well, he is young and inexperienced, and new to Houston. Of course, the main reason they didn't like what he said was that he supported my case and damaged theirs. Thus, the lawyers for BCBS tried to impeach their own witness. I objected because it seemed crazy for the opposing lawyers to impeach their own witness. The judge overruled my objection, and I took an exception to that ruling, so I would have a justification for appeal. Always take exception if you don't agree with a ruling.

Ugh! Despite everything on my side, the judge ruled against me, and I lost that case in his administrative court. It didn't make sense; to this day, I can't explain the judge's decision. This had to be an error. It certainly was not just or justice. Therefore, I wrote an appeal to the three-judge court of appeals in Washington, D.C. Two weeks later (almost by return mail), the appeals court overruled the administrative judge. But, and here is what is very interesting, the appeals court did not remand for a new trial. Instead, they ordered a verdict in my favor and ordered BCBS to pay me with interest, which BCBS did. The amount of money involved was about $32,000, which was a big chunk considering my yearly salary at Baylor College of Medicine was $35,000.

Soon thereafter, the vice president of BCBS visited me at my Methodist Office. He said, "Blue Cross and Blue Shield are afraid of you. Everyone in the main office knows you and fears you."

I told him, "Can we speak frankly? I am sick of BCBS. I know you work for a corrupt organization. I don't know how you can look at yourself in the mirror when you shave in the mornings, knowing what you are going to do at work. I don't want to take care of any of your policyholders. The wasted time can be better spent taking care of other people who need me desperately."

He said, "We can't do that. Each of our insureds is guaranteed access to any doctor they want. We have to consider each case on an individual basis."

Strangely, after that visit, I had no further problem with BCBS. That is, I had no further problems with them until I became a patient and, as a policyholder, needed medical care. In that situation, I had problems galore as you will soon read about at the end of this book, where I discuss my personal experience as a patient, where I get a taste of my own medicine, and where I learn it is better to give than receive. It is better to give care as a doctor than receive care as a patient. There is a world of difference in the power relations. And there is a world of difference between getting paid and paying.

The result in these court cases of me versus BCBS and other insurance companies should convince you that instead of just saluting when the insurance guys say they won't pay, you should exhaust all the internal and external appeals, and then, if they still won't pay, acting as your own attorney, you should sue them. It is easy to do and can be fun. There is nothing to fear except fear itself.

In small money cases, the companies are likely to settle early rather than pay their attorneys. In small money cases, you have the upper hand because you are the attorney and you don't have to pay an attorney the way they do. In big money cases like the Jackson Smith example to follow, it is better to have a real lawyer handle your case.

The Wonderful and Instructive Case of Jackson Smith

Insurance denied payment for my patient, Jackson Smith. He was diagnosed in 1987 by a Birmingham, Alabama neurologist as having amyotrophic lateral sclerosis (ALS). This is a fatal disease, and there was no treatment for it then, and there is still no really effective treatment for it now. ALS is a death sentence.

Jackson read up on his condition and decided he needed a detailed evaluation to prove he had ALS, just in the outside possibility he didn't have ALS but had something else that might be treatable.

Bingo! I proved Jackson had demyelinating neuropathy and didn't have ALS. Severe cases of this disease have been mistaken for ALS. I treated Jackson with Cytoxan, and he improved a little. Then, because Jackson was very weak and getting weaker, I prescribed intravenous gamma globulin.

Jackson's Milwaukee-based insurance company, Time Insurance, Inc., paid for the Cytoxan but balked at the gamma globulin. Gamma globulin is expensive, and I believe that is the reason they refused to pay. But of course, that was not the reason they stated. Instead, they said, "The gamma globulin was experimental and not medically necessary." Always watch out for this ploy. There is a stated reason, but that is often not the real reason. Attack the stated reason. The judges will figure out the real reason.

In a way, they were right. It was experimental, especially considering the policy's very detailed and very exclusive, almost exhaustive definition of experimental. Like a wolf in sheep's clothing, most definitions written by the companies are like an exclusion in disguise, or your insurance company is likely to treat it as one.

The definition of experimental may have the power of life or death, and often, in my experience, has the power to control whether a person diagnosed with cancer can receive the benefits of cutting-edge treatments. I won't bore you with the long and detailed company definition of experimental. Rhonda D. Orin covers it on page 56 of her marvelous book entitled *Making Them Pay: How to Get the Most from Health Insurance and Managed Care.* The major sticking point used by the companies is the almost routine statement at the end of most scientific papers that report clinical breakthrough studies, which says more research is needed. The companies seize on this language. If more research is needed, that confirms that the treatment is still experimental.

Every time you give a patient a medicine, you are experimenting. You don't know for sure what may happen, as every patient is unique. Medical work, in case you haven't figured it out by now, is essentially experimental, uncertain, and, consequently, prone to error. When starting a new treatment, I tell the patient we don't know what is going to happen. "Let's see if this medicine likes you and you like it. One thing is for sure: This medicine will not work if we don't try it."

By the way, no treatment is absolutely necessary. We can always just do nothing and let the disease take its course. Most of our clothing is not necessary. The law requires that we cover our nudity, but that can be done with a newspaper. Strictly speaking, shirts, dresses, shoes, socks, and so forth are not necessary because they do not cover the parts of the body that the law requires to be covered.

In medical care, if we do nothing, some patients will recover. Some will get worse as the disease progresses. Some will die. What happens when the patient is neglected will be good for the insurance company's bottom line and perhaps not so good for the patient.

Be alert!

Watch out for diversionary arguments. When money is involved, insurance companies will try to divert your attention away from the real issue, which usually is money, and onto something fake.

"Medical necessity and experimental" are often fake issues raised because they are trying to see if they can get away with not paying. When Doctor Linda Penno testified before Congress in 1997, she told how managed care organizations profit from complicated contracts, hidden costs, confusing appeals procedures, apathetic members, and various other issues I have already raised and will raise. Here are some excerpts from her testimony:

"First, I exchange my traditional doctor's bag for a health executive's box of tricks. …. We have many ways to eliminate the old, the sick, the disabled, the malignant, the chronic, the risky lifestyles, and many other (sic) who may be a drain on our premium pool."

She then goes on to list the many tricks with item four as follows:

"Fourth, we have our most versatile, authoritative, and profitable tool—our ability to make medical necessary determinations. Empowered with physicians employed by us, we become the final medical authority. Regardless of what any treating physician may want to do, we assume control and practice medicine our way."

Back to Jackson Smith

Result: Because his insurance company refused to pay for his treatment, patient Jackson himself paid. Hooray for Jackson! Boo for Time Insurance.

Yes, Jackson, now 47 years old, footed the bill (over $10,000) for the gamma globulin and recovered his health. Yes, you read correctly. Jackson became normal. Now, Time Insurance was in trouble because the treatment they said was not medically necessary had worked and restored Jackson to normal functioning. He was back to work roofing. He was back working full time, but he was mighty mad about what had happened. Jackson felt his insurance company had screwed him. So, in the great American tradition, he sued his insurance company.

The Federal Court jury, following a five-day trial before Senior U.S. District Court Judge Virgil Pittman, awarded Jackson the $10,000 he paid for the gamma globulin, and gave him $1,250,000 for mental anguish and an additional $3,000,000 in punitive damages.

Gamma globulin is now a standard treatment for demyelinating neuropathy. The companies pay for it. So does Medicare. Or, at least, they had to pay for it for a time, until the companies invented the step-up program. Now, the patients (depending on the specific language in their policy) usually have to take the less expensive and less effective treatment first. If that doesn't work, they may be able to step up to the more expensive, more effective treatment next, provided they are still alive. As for me, give me the best treatment first, regardless of cost. That's how I feel. How about you?

Lesson: Don't step up. Most of us, sooner or later, will be made weak by time and fate. Therefore, make the most of your life now, while there is time and you are in your prime and your youth and blood are warmer. For once having spent your prime, worse and worst times succeed the former. Be prepared right now with the right attitude to fight for what you will need and want in the not-so-great future ahead of you.

This ends what I wanted to tell you about my experiences with insurance as a practicing physician. There are other horror stories I could relate to. You can find them in my book, *Neurology Rounds with the Maverick*. Those of you who are interested in details might profit from the cases of Two Very Sick People and One Not as Sick Administrator (Tableau Three, page 29). There, you will find excellent examples of how insurance tries to eliminate the very sick by claiming the care is a waste of time and money. People pay into the system for decades, but when it is time to get something back, the system balks. Even the rich and famous are not exempt from insurance hassles. Christopher Reeve, in his wonderful best-selling book *Still Me*, discusses his and his wife Dana's ordeals and triumphs on a roll-er-coaster ride to stay alive.

For better or worse, medicine is not an exact science like physics and chemistry. Many times, the practice of medicine is guesswork, as I have already stated. In the case of Jackson Smith, I had a reasonable degree of certainty that the gamma glob-ulin would work because that had been my experience with several other patients who had Jackson's diagnosis.

But we have to face the fact that sometimes a treatment is not really necessary, and sometimes a treatment is really experimental. And therefore, sometimes the insurance company will be right in denying treatment. A case in point was that of Nelene Fox, who had metastatic cancer of the breast. She was 38 and had failed conventional treatments, including surgery and chemotherapy. The cancer had spread to her bones and indicated that she would surely die. Nelene got onto the idea that her only hope was high-dose radiation and bone marrow transplanta-tion. Health Net denied her request for coverage of costs because they said the treatment was experimental and therefore excluded under the terms of her pol-icy. Health Net suggested a second opinion, but Nelene refused and raised the $212,000 she needed through charitable donations. Eight months later, she died. Her husband argued that the delay in treatment caused her death and sued Health Net for bad faith, breach of contract, infliction of emotional and physical damage, and punitive damages. The jury awarded the estate $89 million.

But in this instance, subsequent research proved Health Net was right. The treatment showed no benefit to other patients who had breast cancer and actually worsened their lives. That result must give us pause.

Lesson: Insurance companies are not necessarily always wrong. They are sometimes right, and their denial of coverage may, in some instances, help and not hurt the patient. Every case must be examined in detail to try to arrive at what is right and what is not.

My view is that an outside physician skilled in the care of breast cancer should have been consulted and her/his opinion considered in the final decision to treat or not treat. A second opinion in cases of serious disease and costly and painful treatments is often a good idea.

Before we leave this section, I wanted to show what everyday life was like in my practice, trying to deal with insurance problems.

Background: I employed three clinical nurses and one research nurse. I had a secretary and two insurance clerks. The insurance clerks filled out the insurance forms, and one of them, Martha McKee, was the expert in current procedural technology (CPT) coding. Yes, two full-time employees worked full-time handling the insurance forms. Dale Salazar, my chief clinical nurse, handled the phone calls to insurance companies. Here's how she did it:

First, Dale would have a good lunch and go to the bathroom, and get a cup of coffee. Before she would dial, she would put together some reading material or paperwork because she knew she would be on hold for quite a while. She would get a pen and the insurance log book and take care of everything else that needed to be done, like refilling prescriptions or answering patient questions. She often would smoke a Winston on the third floor of the Methodist Hospital parking garage to adjust her attitude because she knew the calls were going to annoy her. The call would take too long, she would be on hold a lot, and she would deal with numerous people who would not understand her questions and wouldn't help her. She knew she might be on the phone for over an hour and accomplish nothing.

The record of what was done was a key tool in dealing with the companies. Dale would write down the time she called, the number she called, and the number of computerized voices she had to deal with before she got a human to listen. She would note the name of the person she talked to and how long she talked to that person, and how long she had to wait for the person to consult someone or something. Names and titles were important to get if she could get them. In many cases, the people refused to give their name and title and refused to say where they were, though it was often easy to guess that the person was not a primarily English speaker. All these details were noted in the log book because they are needed, because the companies would often "forget" they were called and claim they never were called, or claim they never gave the big OK for admission or treatment. It is difficult for them to make those claims when Dale could say, "at 3:17 on Tuesday, May 5th, I called 800 474 7670 and I was switched from Ophelia Smith, who then after 11 minutes, switched me to Mr. Fortinbras who then consulted a computer program for 5 minutes before turning me over to Doctor Bernardo O'Higgins. Doctor O'Higgins told me he had never heard of Myasthenia Gravis and didn't think it was a real disease. He asked how to spell Myasthenia, and I spelled it for him. He said he had to talk to Doctor Patten directly, so I turned the call and my log notes over to Doctor Patten.

Then, I got on the phone with the insurance company doctor and got right to the point.

Me: "We have a 47-year-old woman with severe myasthenia gravis in crisis. She is in respiratory distress and must be admitted and placed on a respirator until the disease gets under control. This is an emergency. A matter of life or death."

Insurance doctor: "Why can't she be managed as an outpatient?"

Me: "Too sick. That's why."

Insurance doctor: "That doesn't sound serious enough, so I can't certify an admission. You must take care of her as an outpatient."

Me: "Not possible. But since you know so much about this patient, even though you haven't examined her and you didn't, according to nurse Dale, even know how to spell Myasthenia, I want her to go to you for treatment. Give me your street address, and she will arrive by ambulance on a respirator for your excellent care. Many thanks for taking this patient off my hands and good luck to you."

Insurance doctor: "Are you crazy?"

Me: "Nope. Dead serious. Your address, please. And make it fast before the patient tanks."

Insurance doctor: "OK. Preauthorized admission for two days."

Me: "Many thanks. We have recorded your approval."

With all the defeats in court, I thought the companies would have adjusted their general attitude and would have become more tractable.

Nope. I was wrong again. They doubled down on their efforts to delay payment, deny payment, and defend nonpayment. They invented more hoops for the doctors and patients to jump through, and we wasted lots more precious clinical time trying to explain the obvious to the stupid and the intransigent. Routine problems like cataract surgery or retinal detachment are usually handled with dispatch. With unusual diseases like myasthenia gravis, there is usually trouble, lots of it.

The next few years were déjà vu all over again. Many times, I felt like I was rearranging deck chairs on the Titanic. It reached the point that sick people had to pay $20,000 in advance to the hospital to get care because their insurance refused to approve the admission.

Ugh! I was wasting lots of time that I could better spend sleeping or playing the piano, or writing books about the situation.

I loved taking care of patients. I had a vocation as dedicated as any in any religious order. I had pulled many patients out of a deep, dark hole. People who arrived at death's door walked out of the hospital. Think about that. How many chances in a lifetime do you get to cause a cure like that? In my mind, saving a life or reversing dementia was just as important as it would be to make a great medical discovery. For me, the reward of seeing a patient recover was more important than having a high income or making a substantial contribution to medical knowledge. Helping people was a goal in itself. I loved it.

But all good things have to come to an end. I couldn't take the rigamarole anymore and, like so many other physicians, I retired because I was no longer able to continue practicing medicine in a manner that aligned with my convictions regarding the best interests of my patients. But after I retired, I learned a big lesson.

The lesson was that Bernard M. Patten, M.D., was not indispensable. Baylor College of Medicine, Methodist Hospital, and the Muscle and Nerve Clinic all continued to function pretty well without me, though I have a feeling the really complex cases were sent elsewhere or neglected. Wait a second! This might be sour grapes. Maybe I am like Snow White's evil stepmother looking in the mirror and worried that perhaps there are physicians out there better than I was or am. I used to be proud of my many 100+ scientific papers. I still am, but not that much.

Now, looking back, I see things in a different light. My achievements have been more modest than I had thought at the time. My time in the sun is over. Now it's the next generation's turn, though with global warming, the sunlight might not be so benign. The fossil-fuel interests are against measures to mitigate the coming catastrophe of climate change. Their aim is to sow doubt. The same technique was used by the tobacco lobby against banning smoking, an argument used to support your position when you have no evidence in your support, or when the evidence is against you. The doubt arguments are designed to blur the lines between scientific reality and political ideology, treating established facts as debatable opinions. The truth is, conservatives value commerce over the environment. Thus, it is more important than ever that citizens see through the political smokescreens and act accordingly.

Ugh! Have I become a bitter old man? Sometimes I think the human race has had a frontal lobotomy. Looking at global politics and the arms race and nuclear proliferation with numerous nameless missiles planted on the soils of Russia, China, and America's midwestern farmland, with more to come, all poised to fly out at a moment's notice and engineered to ignite cities at the temperature of the sun, 10,000 degrees Fahrenheit, makes me think of school boys in the playground. I'm having trouble deciding whether the boys in charge function at third- or fourth-grade levels. What's your view?

Sigmund Freud, after practicing psychotherapy for decades in Vienna, believed that the human race was doomed. In the very long term, this is inevitable, after all. It bothers me to sleep that my grandchildren and descendants may or will suffer the decline that ending the human race will involve.

Nevertheless, it is still my informed opinion that modern medicine doesn't have the time, knowledge, or skill to diagnose or treat rare illnesses like inner membrane carnitine palmityl transferase deficiency or, say, Alexander's disease of Glial Fibrillary Acid Protein mutations. Such patients who are unlucky enough to have a non-routine illness are stuck and out of luck.

Since my retirement, conditions for physicians have gotten worse. There's much more paperwork. For every hour spent seeing patients, according to the American Medical Association, the average doctor now spends two hours doing administrative tasks. A primary driver of the paperwork is, believe it or not, the electronic health record (EHR). The electronic health record was supposed to eliminate the paper-based tracking system and make patients' health records easier to access. That was in theory. In practice, the opposite was true. The main focus became documentation (and I believe padding) for regulators to see and for billing insurance. To handle the increased demands, doctors had to work on their charts for long hours at home at night when they should be having fun with their family or reading medical journals or both. Doctors began cutting office hours, and hence the long wait periods and the rush to get the present patient out to see the next in line. Very bad—all this is very bad. The doctor-patient relation needs time to establish trust. One of the great rewards of medicine in the golden era was getting to know the patients on a personal basis. Alas, much of the personal service that used to exist is now out the window. People I talk to at cocktail parties don't even know the name of the doctor who did their cataract surgery or who repaired their retinal detachment. That proves the problem works both ways. The doctor doesn't know the patient, and the patient doesn't know the doctor.

The other problem that I have heard from those still in the trenches is that corporations have bought the practices and now dictate how medicine is to be practiced, and in many cases, the dictates are not in the patient's best interest. My son-in-law says, "Many aspects of the doctor's professional life are controlled, and it's all about money. The doctor is not in charge. Approvals from the powers-that-be have to be obtained to order tests and to prescribe treatments."

The fastest-growing physician group in Harris County, Texas, is the retired physicians' association, and I know why. My problems were general and not particular. Those doctors (many of them anyway) couldn't take it either, so they left the profession.

Something has to be done. Some countervailing power has to be mobilized to exert control for the public good and for the welfare of patients and doctors. One countervailing power and a way forward is through your congressman. Until Congress takes the problems seriously and provides modern laws to protect you and your family, you are on the spot.

The legal system and courts offer some hope, but not much. My small victories in court don't amount to a hill of beans compared to the enormity of the problems and what is happening all around America. Still, occasionally, there is some good news.

For instance, on January 8, 2025, Texas Medicine notified me that the landmark antitrust settlement against BCBS was granted preliminary approval. Physicians, myself included, may now file a claim in a $2.8 billion settlement fund given approval by a U.S. District Court involving Blue Cross and Blue Shield. The settlement is expected to bring substantial changes, including accountability, streamlining claims processing, and reducing administrative burdens. The settlement involves all BCBS entities, as well as the Blue Cross Blue Shield Association, and will require BCBS to "invest millions in system improvements to address widespread issues currently affecting providers."

Texas Medical Association President G. Ray Callas finds the settlement encouraging. He said, "No matter what insurance plan it is or what health plan it is, we definitely need transparency and streamlining related to claims processing and… authorizations to make sure that physicians are being paid timely and appropriately."

Note: This litigation was initiated in 2000 and joined by the Texas Medical Association a year later. The mills of justice grind exceedingly slow. Meanwhile, for 24 years, BCBS continued to abuse patients and doctors. In my view, the settlement is probably just a fraction of what BCBS made in profits by their bad behavior.

The suit, by the way, accused 10 of the nation's major private health plans of conspiring to delay and reduce payments to clinicians and hospitals by down-coding claims (sound familiar?) and using intimidation tactics during contract negotiations. The lawsuit was brought under the Racketeer Influenced and Corrupt Organizations Act (RICO).

See. It wasn't just me. Others, including a federal judge, think Blue Cross and Blue Shield is a corrupt organization.

Here's the latest from *Texas Medicine Today*, the official bulletin of the Texas Medical Association: February 12, 2025. "More than one in five claims denied in Texas by non-group qualified health plans. A study of health plans available through HealthCare.gov shows one in five claims nationwide were denied—with Texas ranking among the top five states for in network denials. …UnitedHealth Group, with the top market share, was shown in the study to have the most denials.

"In network denials for insurers operating in Texas, per the study, included:

- United Health Group, 33%
- Health Care Services Corporation, which includes Blue Cross and Blue Shield of Texas (BCBSTX), 29%
- Molina Healthcare, 26%
- Elevance Health, 23%
- CVS, 21%
- Scott & White, 19%
- Harris, 18%

- Oscar Health, 17% and
- Centene, 14%

…19% of in-network claims and 37% of out-of-network claims were denied by insurers.…With premiums also on the rise…patients are paying more per month with increased denials of service."

Full text of this bulletin should be available to you on texmed.org

Conclusion: Corporate greed is documented again. Patients pay more for health insurance but get less. Remember, the denial rate is merely the tip of the iceberg. Often, there are other problems with the claims. With each claim, there may come associated mean abuses of doctors and policyholders, which you probably know by now include low pay, slow pay, and no pay.

Goethe: "Allwissend bin ich nicht; doch viel ist mir bewisst."

German: I do not know everything, but many things I understand.

Here is the next thing I understand. Primary care is under attack. Primary care in the United States has traditionally led the delivery of preventive services, a high-value function for maximizing public health. Now, the already weak system faces a new source of disruption: functional primary care groups are being acquired by private investors and large Fortune 500 companies, such as Walmart, Amazon.com, CVS, Walgreens, and UnitedHealth Group. Some of these investors and companies are already treating these practices as tradeable commodities rather than critical elements in a national health system. The resulting effects on the functioning of what remains of primary care in the United States forecast stormy weather and deserve careful scrutiny by policymakers.

Section B—The Modern Scene—Experience as a Patient

"No memory of having starred makes up for later disregard or keeps the end from being hard." Robert Frost

Here begins my modern medical encounters as a patient, during which I often get a taste of my own medicine and lament the passing of aspects of the golden age.

As a patient, I quickly learned that the doctor and the patient are not on the same wavelength and certainly do not have the same equivalent status. The view is entirely different when you are making rounds with your entourage of nurses, residents, students, and fellows, while you are standing there at the bedside looking down at a patient—that view is completely different from when you are lying in the bed looking up at the doctor. From the change in perspective, I learned multiple lessons. If I could go back, I would do my practice differently from what I did. Life doesn't give us that chance. Too bad! The best I can do is tell you what happened and hope you doctors and patients can learn from it and do better than I did.

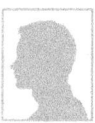

I GET CATARACT SURGERY

MODERN ENCOUNTER ONE: I GET CATARACT SURGERY

◆ ◆ ◆

March 1, 2023, at 6 AM, I reported to the Surgi Center in Webster, Texas, for the removal of the cataract in my right eye and the insertion of a plastic lens in its place. Ethel, my wife of 60 years, came with me because it was likely that after surgery and anesthesia, I would be in no shape to drive.

Getting up early was a pain, and so was not eating breakfast. The Surgi Center had a long list of instructions sent to me via email. Forms take the place of personal, friendly contact and avoid having to spend time answering questions.

No food or water after midnight was part of the deal. In addition, I had to fill in pages and pages of health information in order to get something called a Surgipass that would permit me to get service at the Surgi Center.

Filling out the forms was annoying and took 32 minutes of my precious time. Anytime someone hands you a form, they are likely to be wasting your life for their own benefit and purposes. The main idea of the health form was, I suppose, to have something on record that they could show that would tend to prove they did a complete medical history. In case of a lawsuit, such a document might help their defense. My hope was that someone would actually read and understand the health form, especially the part about my severe allergy to aspirin.

The main idea I needed to get across on the form was that I was severely allergic to aspirin. One aspirin would throw me into anaphylactic shock with severe swelling on my face and difficulty breathing. This has happened twice in my lifetime and almost killed me both times. I didn't want to have it happen again. My allergy cross-reacts with the nonsteroidal anti-inflammatory agents, so they too are contraindicated in my case.

This new form was annoying because I had already filled out a similar form for my eye doctor, Kai Chu, and for my personal concierge doctor, Donna Sue Dolle. The new form was a duplication of previous forms that I believed were unnecessary. Care, I think ruefully, is replaced by forms and printed handouts. Too bad!

Other complaints: to get on the surgery schedule, I had to stop wearing my contact lenses for six weeks and, instead, wear very thick, heavy eyeglasses, which I hate. And there were eye tests I had to endure weeks before surgery in order to get the proper measurement for the plastic lens. One of those tests involved ultrasound of the eye with measurement of focal length and corneal curvature. That special test cost me $600 because BCBS refused to pay. BCBS refused to pay because "the test was not covered." When I asked why it was not covered, I was told, "Because it is not covered." That was my first lesson about BCBS: They were very good at tautology (needless repetition) and very good at denial of claims. My private doctor, Donna Sue Donne, also had to fill out a health form certifying, in her opinion I would survive anesthesia and surgery, and she had to fax a report of my recent electrocardiogram. Having my own private doctor like Donna Sue is a great blessing and a wonderful tool in dealing with the rigmarole.

Lesson: Get a private concierge physician (if you can afford one) and grapple her to your soul with hoops of steel.

I guess there were legitimate medical reasons for some of these forms, but the dark side of me thought most of it was to protect the doctors and the Surgi Center from lawsuits.

In the old days, I breezed into surgery to do the operation. Today was different. I was one of the common herd, one of many people waiting.

The waiting room was filled. I counted 52, but I am sure some were not patients. Some were just relatives there to help. There were no children. Everyone looked over 50, and many, like myself (age 83), looked way over the hill. Some had actually brought food and were eating, and others were actually nodding off. One man had stretched out on a table and was sleeping. He must have had prior experience because he knew how to take advantage of wait time.

I checked in with the unsmiling admissions secretary and was handed six more pages of forms.

"Oh, no. More forms. Does anyone ever read them?"

She smiled and said, "I don't know, I've only worked here three years."

"What the devil do you do with all this paperwork?" I asked.

"I don't know. I think they are photographed and stored digitally in a computer somewhere."

"Why?"

"I don't know. That's how we do things."

"After the forms are returned to you, does anyone read them?"

"I haven't seen anyone read them, but someone elsewhere might read them, but I doubt it. It's just routine."

Conclusion: Seldom are the forms explained; seldom are they even read.

I glanced over the forms. These were notices about my legal rights and also forms for me to exonerate the center if anything went wrong. Again, I had to fill in my first name, middle name, last name, date of birth, social security number, nearest kin with phone number, whom to notify in an emergency or in case of death, and, most importantly, I had to fill out a section about my insurance carrier. The insurance carrier question was about who was going to pay, and I had to sign a paper that I would pay if insurance didn't. Never ever did I ask any patient how they would pay. That is a modern thing. And it seemed to me insurance was the coin of the realm because the secretary told me she had to copy my insurance card and call the company to confirm coverage.

"Why? Rachel at Doctor Chu's office confirmed my coverage two weeks ago. And so did the Surgi Center last week."

She shook her head. "Have to confirm today. It's the rule."

"Why is it the rule?"

"I'm not sure. But I have to do it."

"Do you have to confirm for everyone?"

"No. Just some companies. Blue Cross is one."

We waited an hour. The room gradually emptied as a nurse called the patients to the door to the actual operating area. Some patients came out, and their relatives helped them leave.

After a while, at about 10:15, my wife and I were almost alone in the waiting room, so I asked the secretary what was up. She told me I was still on hold because they were still trying to confirm the insurance. No one was answering the call at BCBS. "Not to worry. This is routine."

Finally, the secretary called me over. "You are confirmed and preapproved, and preauthorized for cataract surgery. The nurse will call you into the operating area soon."

Twenty minutes later, I was called. I was beginning to learn that "soon" in medical lingo had a very different meaning from what is usually understood.

Now I was with a nurse in a small side room. She spoke with a British accent. She is from Liverpool. Her job was to review my medical history and prepare me for surgery. She handed me another long legal document in fine print, which I couldn't read because I left my reading glasses in the waiting room with Ethel.

The nurse assured me it was just routine, stating that I knew the risks of the surgery and anesthesia, namely, among other things, blindness, paralysis, and death.

"But I had already signed one such form outside at the admission desk."

"That form relieved the Surgi Center of responsibility; this form protects the surgeon and the anesthesiologist."

I do understand the reasons for the forms. Health care providers are worried about being sued, particularly since the courts have ruled that the patient must be fully informed of all the risks and alternatives. Those lawsuits—the MedMals—medical malpractice suits, never were problems in the golden era. When I first was in practice, my yearly medical malpractice premium was $100. In the second year of practice, I got a letter from the company apologizing because they raised the yearly malpractice premium to $125. No kidding. That's all I paid. Now I will bet the surgeon and anesthesiologist pay much more, maybe even $100,000 a year.

My father was a lawyer. All his advice and my training forbade me from signing without reading and understanding. I told the nurse that no one had really explained anything to me. The only thing I got handed so far was multiple forms.

The startled nurse frowned and stood. She announced, "I have to get a doctor to handle things when a patient gets difficult."

So, I signed. What else was there to do? It seemed useless to do anything else. I knew from experience that disturbing a well-oiled machine can result in disaster. My inner voice said, "Don't rock the boat."

Right?

The nurse shuffled a few more papers and asked if I was allergic to anything.

God damn!

My Surgipass forms had not been read! The very key concern of mine had not been noticed, much less addressed. After my explanation, the nurse put a big white armband on my left wrist, which read in big red letters: ALLERGIC TO ASPERIN (sic). She meant *Aspirin*—she couldn't even spell it correctly.

She then assisted me into an open space where I was subject to the final indignity. They took all my clothes away and gave me a skimpy piece of cloth that opened wide in back, exposing my butt. I felt like I was being treated like a baby, and I felt just as helpless. Then, they put me in a bed and hooked up a whole bunch of monitors: blood pressure, breathing, blood oxygen, electrocardiogram (EKG).

Ugh! I read my own EKG, which was prominently displayed in brilliant green on the monitor: It showed first-degree AV block. I hope no one else notices, otherwise they might cancel my surgery. AV block is a prolongation of the electrical impulse from the atrium of the heart to the ventricles. The prolongation of the impulse suggests that at some time in the future, I may need a pacemaker. I hope not soon. I hope not ever.

Lying in bed in a surgical suite was a new experience for me. I had been in similar rooms many times, but in a different position. In those days, I was the surgeon. I was in command. I was there looking down at my obedient, humble, and usually helpless patient who was in bed. Now, the patient was me! I have been literally stripped of my power, my dignity. But what could I do? I had to continue with the ritual. Otherwise, Too-da-loo and no dice. If the cataract was not fixed, I would have to continue suffering from poor vision and glare. Besides, I had already invested too much time and energy preparing for this event and adventure. Alia jacta est. Latin: The die was cast.

It was getting late and approaching lunchtime. Man, was I hungry. Yes, I was concerned about eating and wondered when I would get to eat. Probably not for quite a while. Eating has always been a big item for me.

I was also concerned about the anesthesiologist. As a doctor, I knew horror stories about anesthesia mistakes. A surgeon injected one tonsil, and the six-year-old patient slumped over dead. The student nurse had loaded the syringe with cocaine instead of Novocain, the usual local anesthetic at that time. Some patients given a preoperative injection of morphine never made it to the operating room. Was it an overdose or an allergic reaction? We'll never know. Visions of that movie, *Coma*, raced through my head, where the gas carbon monoxide was substituted for oxygen, producing irreversible brain damage.

The anesthesiologist came and told me he would use mild sedation because I was old and might not survive more general anesthesia. That was not encouraging. He told me the main risk was not from the surgery, which was trivial, but from the anesthesia itself, which could cause lots of problems, including death. By the way, he asked, "Are you allergic to anything?" This question did not instill confidence. He hadn't read my Surgiform. Naturally, I explained, after pointing to the arm band, my major concern. He read the arm band, but he didn't seem to notice that aspirin was spelled wrong.

Next, the anesthesia nurse came. His name was Billy, and he was the first person who actually introduced himself and told me his name. He said he was going to do the anesthesia.

"While under supervision, I hope."

Billy smiled and nodded yes. Again, I was asked if I was allergic to anything. Again, I was informed about the risk of death. Billy asked, "If you have a cardiac arrest, do you wish to be resuscitated?"

"No thanks."

"So, no code for you. Is that right?"

"Yes, no code."

Finally, Kai Chu, my ophthalmologist, arrived. At first, I didn't recognize her. She looked so different, dressed in an operating outfit and mask. She explained what was going to happen and what she would do. She answered my questions without hesitation or condescension. Hurray! At last, a compassionate doctor. This whole thing must be routine for her, but it wasn't for me, and I appreciated her courtesy in explaining what was what. I told her I trusted her explicitly and implicitly. She thanked me and said I was next and would be taken into the operating room soon.

There it was again, that medical "soon." It felt like a century went by, but it probably was only twenty minutes until Billy arrived. At last, it was time for surgery.

"Ready, Doctor Patten?"

Oh God, this guy is a gem. He is the first person, besides Doctor Kai Chu, who addressed me as doctor and who knew my name.

"Billy, I changed my mind. Full code, please."

"Right, oh, Doc. It's going in. Have a good sleep."

And then, I knew nothing. I didn't think, I couldn't see, I couldn't feel anything, I didn't know I was alive. I couldn't move my arms, legs, or anything.

This must be what death is like. You don't know anything. You can't move and you can't see or hear or feel or smell or taste or think. The dead probably don't even know they are dead. Death, I have a hunch, is just like general anesthesia, except that from anesthesia, some people wake up. The dead never wake. Never! "The undiscovered country from whose borne no traveler returns puzzles the will and makes us rather bear the ills we have than fly to others that we know not of." Shakespeare.

With one simple injection in a matter of minutes, the person that I had been was no longer existing. Just prior to the injection, I had been a subject and a center of a clinical reality as a patient. But all of a sudden, time had stopped. The person that was "me" ceased to exist. Where my personality went, I know not. I think it simply became extinct, sort of like a candle flame when it goes out. The flame doesn't go anywhere; it just ceases to exist. The idea that the flame goes anywhere is a trick of language. It doesn't go anywhere. It simply becomes extinct. The flame stopped being a flame, the way under anesthesia, I stopped being a person, stopped being me. My conscious self and my unconscious self are made up of the electrical activity of over 100 billion neurons. I am both my conscious self and my unconscious self. Some drug erased half of myself, the conscious part.

What part of me remained after anesthesia was merely an object. Stretched on the table, I was a piece of furniture in a repair shop. For those who surround me, the masked actors; all there was of me was my body. My personality, my real conscious self, what is considered the real "me," was withdrawn, no longer present.

Next time I have cataract surgery, if there is a next time, I shall insist on being fully awake so I can know what's going on and entertain the group with jokes and interesting stories and be my real true self all during the procedure.

OK. Let's skip to the future for a short follow-up:

Left eye cataract replaced under local anesthesia. I was awake throughout and joked with the staff and Doctor Chu as they were working. The cost was nicely covered by Medicare A and B with no hassle. The way this works is wonderful. The government contracts with hospitals and doctors on the amount of payment for various items. The contract amount becomes the agreed cost, and the government pays 100% of the hospitalization and 80% of the physician's fee. So, if the physician's regular fee is $5,000 (for example) for cataract surgery, Medicare Part B might allow $800 as per contract. Therefore, the patient only pays $160, and the government pays the rest. In my view, we should have Medicare like this working for everyone. A special form of insurance is available to pay for the gap of 20% if you wish to pay the premiums. Medicare Advantage programs are somewhat different from traditional Medicare. They usually have geographic limits, meaning you must get your care in a prescribed area, and they also usually have personnel limits, meaning you must get your care from a physician enrolled in their network. Thus, with Medicare Advantage, you might have trouble if you live in Houston going to Cleveland Clinic for your heart surgery or going to the one of three expert physicians in the world in New York City who knows about and can treat myoadenylate deficiency or some other unusual or rare disease.

Back to the narration about modern encounter one, cataract surgery.

I awoke. The recovery room was bright and clean. Two nurses, a cute young redhead and a more mature blond, hovered over me, all smiles. The redhead was holding my hand. It was a nice sensation and confirmed that the anesthesia had not damaged my brain too much.

"All over, Doctor Patten. Are you in any pain?"

"Nope. No Pain."

Shortly, Doctor Chu turned up, all smiles too. She said everything went well. Of course, I was not reassured, though a lay person might have been. I have seen too many patients given false assurances. So, I know better. I have been around and no longer believe doctors are infallible. Time, and time alone, will tell if everything went alright.

Clair Harman, my son's acting teacher, said her neurosurgeon, Ed Murphy, assured her that he had removed the brain cancer completely. I doubt that is what Ed told her, but I would bet that is what she wanted to hear. She had a glioblastoma, a cancer no one survives. I had to set her straight and urge her to prepare for departure.

It was the end of the trail. Several months later, she died from a recurrence. Another patient was told the sections of the tumor removed at surgery were read as benign, which they were. But several weeks later, on reexam, the reverse was true (now the same tissue read as malignant), and ultimately that patient died of her cancer.

The reverse is also true. I have known patients and their families who had been advised that their prognosis was hopeless, and yet the patient survived. A patient was told he had pancreatic cancer and only three months to live. After six months, he consulted another doctor. The cancer diagnosis was wrong. He had an inflammatory disease of the pancreas (pancreatitis) that was mistaken for a cancer. The pancreatitis went away by itself.

And then there was Evy, who had ALS (amyotrophic lateral sclerosis), a fatal disease, fully confirmed by me after an exhaustive work-up, and who was in respiratory distress at the time I told her to plan her funeral. Two years later, she returned for re-examination, claiming the disease was gone, and by God, it was. Was her recovery a miracle? I don't think so. But on the other hand, I can't explain it. She said she knew the ALS was just an excuse to get out of the terrible job (she hated) as a hospital director. Having left her job, she then had time to travel and realized she had discovered her true self—that she was bisexual and happy paying for sex and friendship. According to her, her body no longer needed a sickness as an excuse not to work, and therefore, because the sickness was no longer useful to her or needed, it cured itself, and the ALS disappeared.

I looked around the recovery room. I was seeing a little better with my right eye even without glasses, so I guessed everything did go OK.

Doctor Chu said she would check me in her office at three this afternoon just to make sure everything was right. I like doctors who follow up on their work. That is very important, and it is one way they learn what they did right and what they did wrong.

I asked my two nurses, "Who owns the Surgi Center?"

They shrugged their shoulders and said in unison, "We don't know. Probably some doctors."

"Well, who pays you?"

More shrugged shoulders. "Don't know," said the blonde. We just get a check from the center."

"How about something to eat?"

"Not here. That's a no-no. We'll get your clothes and a wheelchair. Sounds like you're ready to go. Blood O2 is 98, and EKG is normal."

My EKG still showed AV block, but I wasn't about to tell them or anyone that it wasn't normal. Sometimes it pays to keep your mouth shut.

"I don't want a wheelchair. I am able to walk."

"Wheelchair is a must. Routine."

Wow! I learned a lot from my first modern medicine encounter. Among other things, I learned that it is much more difficult to be a patient than I ever imagined. There are multiple inconveniences and annoyances.

First, you have to get to the venue for care. In my case, the Surgi Center was a half-hour away, and it took a half-hour to get back home. Doctor Chu's office is a half-hour away, and that means a half-hour back. Adding the numbers, we get two hours of travel time on the day of surgery.

But that was nothing compared to what my patients had to endure. My practice lasted 22 years at Methodist Hospital. During that time, patients came from New York, Ohio, Michigan, Alabama, Texas, Louisiana, California, Mexico, Peru, Argentina, Taiwan, Paris, London, Venice, Malaysia, South Korea, Thailand, and even Russia. I am ashamed to admit that I never ever gave it a second thought about the time, energy, and money that these patients spent to travel to consult me. For two decades, it was routine for the Canadian Health Service to pay for transportation and the hospital care of Canadian citizens who had muscle diseases. The hospital and I never failed to get paid, and there was never a question about the bill. The South American trade was very interesting and included the presidents of countries, Peruvian Generals, and wealthy businessmen. Usually, the patients from South America brought presents. The General from Peru brought a pre-Columbian vase and seeds for giant corn plants that grew to 16 feet. The kernels in the cobs were as big as my thumb. Often, the Mexicans tipped me with gold coins. Chinese patients gave Ming Dynasty antiques or what they said were from the Ming Dynasty. I handled the Chinese because my Mandarin is pretty good. Dale Salazar, my chief clinical nurse, spoke fluent Spanish and made those patients feel at home.

I would like to go back in time, knowing now what the plight of patients really is like, and change the way I practiced by being more sympatico. I won't go back in time because it would change the space-time continuum. But in a moment of weakness, perhaps I would tell my young Bernie self to put all his money into Apple Computer stock in the 1980s. That way, I would now have a very well-funded retirement plan and wouldn't have to fight insurance companies for payments.

Come to think of it, my car trip to the Surgi Center was no big deal compared to the travel travails that my own patients had to suffer. I made a mental note to bring Doctor Chu something, probably one of my books.

Parking at the Surgi Center was inconvenient. We had to park far from the entrance and walk in. The parking at Doctor Chu's League City office will be easier.

Second problem at the Surgi Center—ridiculous waiting. Think of those people, not only in America but around the world, who are wasting their precious lives waiting and waiting and waiting. Two patients at M.D. Andersen Cancer Hospital (Glen and Judy Grace) told me they routinely waited several hours past their appointment time each and every clinic visit. The waiting stopped when Judy died of mesothelioma.

Waiting is one of the worst aspects of being a patient. Waiting in drab outpatient waiting areas, waiting for appointments, waiting for them to wheel you into the operating room, waiting for the results of tests and scans. When doctors are faced with piles of paperwork and extra work on the bane of their existence, the EHR (the electronic health record), it is difficult for them to keep in mind that each result has an anxious patient attached to it. That's one of the many great advantages of having a concierge doctor. Doctor Dolle routinely sends a message as soon as the lab results are in and writes about her interpretation and advice.

Back to the Adventure at the Surgi Center

Conclusion: long waits = not good. Adjustments are needed.

In my clinic, I was never more than 15 minutes behind —except once, when I had to leave to save the life of an engineer whose subdural was about to kill him. All doctors should follow my example out of decent respect for patients. Staying on time requires discipline, mainly of the doctor and medical staff, but sometimes also of the patients, some of whom talk too much or demand extra time.

One day, a lawyer from Baton Rouge arrived late and wanted to be seen. I explained I couldn't fit him in without inconveniencing the many patients who arrived on time. He complained to the office administrator, but that got nowhere because in the golden age I, the doctor, was in charge and had the final say-so. That lawyer filed a lawsuit against me, asking for reimbursement of $176 that he said it cost him to come to Houston.

Two weeks later, his sister came to talk to me. She said, "Henry did that to everyone. He was always late and insisted on being served nevertheless. You were the only person who ever stood up to him. You don't have to worry about the lawsuit. He wouldn't be around anymore. Last week, he died of a heart attack."

After the unnecessary wait at the Surgi Center, there was a more important problem. The failure of the system to read my health form and recognize I had a very serious allergy to aspirin.

Ah, I crossed to the other side. I have to stop complaining. I have become just another patient, another old man in for cataract surgery. I had no right to claim I needed or deserved special treatment. They didn't read my Surgipass. They probably never read anyone's. But I'm a doctor. I have been around, and I can partially compensate for the neglect. But what of the general public? This kind of slipshod approach can have dire consequences.

Health records should be read and understood. Allergies should be noted.

In my day, I have seen plenty of nurses in action. I can tell right away when they are burned out and just going through the motions. That seemed to be the problem with the intake nurse. And let's face it, many nurses are not only burned out; they are not very smart. And some are just plain stupid. I recall doing a consult at Hermann Hospital. The patient had dermatomyositis, my specialty. But the charge nurse told me to forget the consult. The patient was bleeding to death. And he was. There was bright red blood coming out of his ass. Four intravenous lines were running in. Three lines were pumping blood, trying to keep up with the gastrointestinal bleeding. By instinct, I examined the fourth line. It was heparin! The patient was getting an anticoagulant while bleeding! Unbelievable but true. The shocked nurse said she couldn't stop the heparin, but she knew it should be stopped. At last, a smart nurse! But she had to get the doctor in charge to order the change. We waited, but the attending physician was not answering his page.

I volunteered to stop the heparin, but the nurse said I can't because I am only the consultant. Of course, I went right over and shut off the heparin. The bleeding soon stopped, and the patient and I knew I had saved his life. Unthinking nurses and Nazi nurses are a plague. Good nurses are pure gold. Doctors should answer emergency pages right away.

Hospital mistakes are common. Errors in medication, diet, and procedures occur. Sometimes the surgeon will operate at the wrong spinal level or on the wrong eye. I know of a neurosurgeon who removed normal brain tissue instead of the arteriovenous malformation he was aiming for. Another surgeon operated on the wrong side of the brain for a brain tumor. He removed normal brain instead. That mistake caused lots of legal trouble for him, but he did not lose his hospital privileges.

One last rant: The forms that I thought were amusing were the ones that notified me of my special legal rights as a patient, among these the right to ask questions, the right to be fully informed, and the right to be treated with respect and dignity. And beyond these forms, there were those notices on the walls (even in the men's room) declaring that patients are treated with dignity and respect. Despite all that, we patients were still seen as an underclass. Improving the hospital environment has a long way to go. If patients were really treated with dignity and respect, there would be no need for all those notices. And no need for all those guest relation departments to handle complaints. If patients were treated with respect and dignity, there would be a lot less wasted time.

Here ends the narrative of my first modern encounter.

What was good? Not so good?

What was bad and what was ugly?

I have my views.

Reader, you decide.

Compare and contrast my experience with your own experiences and those of the golden age of medicine.

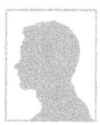

MODERN ENCOUNTER TWO

FOLLOW UP EXAM AT DOCTOR CHU'S OFFICE

MODERN ENCOUNTER TWO: FOLLOW UP EXAM AT DOCTOR CHU'S OFFICE

◆ ◆ ◆

No problem with parking and not much wait time until I was called by the technician. But there was a problem, a serious problem that I noticed on the drive down. I couldn't see the stop signs or the traffic lights with my right eye. Good that Ethel was driving and not me. In fact, I couldn't see a blessed thing with my right (operated) eye. That eye was blind! But I wasn't panicked. The sheet of papers that I had agreed to did mention the risk of blindness. So, more or less, I accepted my fate. I took a chance, and things didn't work out. I had waited until that eye was really bad. That is, in my own mind, I thought it was a good idea to wait until I had nothing much to lose with the operation.

The tech measured intraocular pressure and was relieved it was normal. She confirmed that I was blind. I couldn't see the big E on the Snellen chart. I couldn't even see the chart or the wall on which the chart letters were displayed. She held fingers in front of my right eye. Again nothing.

My left eye was OK at 20/20. That was a relief. "In the kingdom of the blind, the one-eyed man is king." I am quoting Erasmus, the Dutch Scholar (1465-1536). I was pretty sure I could adjust to having only one eye. Lots of other people, including some of my friends, have that disability. One of them is even a licensed airplane pilot.

"Why can't I see?"

"I can't say. Doctor Chu will see you soon."

The tech then led us to another waiting room where we sat waiting with about a dozen other patients. After about half an hour, we were put in a room and waited for Doctor Chu, who took a look at the computer and then examined my eyes with the slit lamp. She said everything looked good. "Continue the drops. Corneal edema (excess fluid in tissue) should clear in a few days."

"Doctor Chu, how many did you do today?"

"Eight cataracts, including you."

My brother, who is a cataract surgeon, explained that Chu probably had to use a lot of ultrasound energy to remove a very hard cataract. The extra energy "annoyed" the cornea and produced corneal edema. Corneal edema was making the eye blind. Time and the steroid drops should improve things. Later on, Jim warned me that the posterior lens capsule might get opaque because of the energy used on the cataract. That would require laser surgery to make a hole that I could see through. Jim also added that he does not do high myope patients like me. "Too risky! With the high myopes like you, it is much harder to get a good result. Those patients are a pain in the ass, so I send them to Houston! Relax. Kai Chu is the best in Houston. You are in good hands."

The right eye was blind for the next three days. On day four, in the evening, when Ethel was putting in the drops, I thought I saw a vague outline of her head, but I couldn't see any details of her face. The next day, I saw much more, and within two more days, I was seeing well with that eye. The plastic lens inserted was focused for reading. So, I now had what is called monovision: The left eye geared for distant and the right for close-up. I got a set of glasses for driving with the right lens a minus two to give me 20/20 for distance on the right and the left lens plain glass. The new glasses cost $1,000. It was worth it to see normally while driving. The whole patchwork treatment to get rid of the cataract was worth the suffering I endured. I was now seeing better than ever. Colors were vivid and vibrant and beautiful, especially the blues. Little did I know at the time that more trouble, big trouble concerning the surgery, was headed my way.

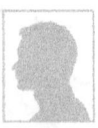

MODERN ENCOUNTER THREE

THE BILL ARRIVES; INSURANCE BALKS

MODERN ENCOUNTER THREE: THE BILL ARRIVES; INSURANCE BALKS

◆ ◆ ◆

May 14, 2023 found me in Macon, Georgia, to help my grandson Jorell celebrate his graduation from Mercer College with a degree in supply chain management, an academic subject that did not exist in my day. CVS sent me an email reminder that I was due to pick up the prescription for Tamsulosin HCl 0.4 mg capsules for my prostate problem. The CVS in Macon had the prescription on file, but the pharmacist wanted to know who was going to pay.

Me: "My insurance, Express Scrips Medicare (PDP) for UT Care, usually pays almost everything."

Pharmacist: "Your insurance has been cancelled."

This was the first time I had heard anything like this. It shook me. Must be a mistake.

Me: "Cancelled? When?"

Pharmacist: "March 1, 2023, at 10 AM."

Me: "That's impossible. That was the day I had cataract surgery. They wouldn't cancel me when I was under the knife. Besides, I was preapproved, and the surgery was preauthorized."

Pharmacist: "Definitely cancelled. The prescription part of your insurance was terminated on April 30. That's what they said."

Me: "Terminated?"

Pharmacist: "They said terminated. I put some sugar on it, saying it was cancelled. Are you picking up the TAM or not?"

An hour later, I got the prescription and paid the full amount. The next day, I called my health adviser at Blue Cross and Blue Shield. There was no question about it: The insurance cancelled me on March 1, the day of surgery, and the pharmacy part on the last day of April. This was done without my knowledge or consent. They didn't even have the courtesy of notifying me directly.

On the phone, I worked through the computers and finally got to three health advisors, each of whom conveyed the same message in no uncertain terms that the cancellation was not the plan's problem. The cancellation was my problem, and insurance can be cancelled any time for any reason, and for no reason whatsoever. The message was: "Tough luck, Patten," although they didn't state it that way. They clearly thought that a private company has the legal right to cancel anytime they wish, even if you continued to pay the premiums.

Doctor Peeno's testimony before the Senate now rang true. Remember: She said, "We have many ways to eliminate the old, the sick, the disabled, the malignant, the chronic, the risky lifestyles, and any other who may be a drain on our premium pool."

That was it: I was being eliminated as a drain on the premium pool, probably because, as an 83-year-old gomer, I would likely, in the future, require lots more care. The reason this cancellation sounds unfair is because it is unfair. It is just another unfair trick to maximize profits at the expense of schmucks like me. Longevity does not fit into the business model of our current health insurance system.

Here is a copy of the letter I sent to Richard Blumenthal, the chair of the United States Senate subcommittee on health.

Dear Senator Blumenthal:

Some computer program terminated our long-held insurance because we are old and now need insurance coverage. Here's the details:

My UT Select identification number is UTSOAH9DM14Q

Group number 071778

Coverage date 09/01/22

On May 14, the CVS pharmacist told me my insurance was terminated. On May 15, I called my BCBS Health Advocate at 1-888-882-2034, who told me my insurance was terminated March 1, the day of my cataract surgery, and my drug program was terminated April 30. Three people said on the phone that my insurance was terminated by a computer program and not by any human being. They were not able to explain why it was terminated because the information was not available to them. Evidently, there was an algorithm program that kicked in. The program is a commercial secret, so they don't have access to it. Needless to say, I don't have access either.

May 19, 2023, I got a letter, dated May 5, from Express Scrips which says, "We received your request to disenroll from Express Scrips Medicare (PDP) for UT CARE." That is an incorrect statement, so I called Member Customer Service at 1-800-860-7849 and spoke to a computer and three humans who could not explain why the letter said I requested disenrollment when I didn't. They said they had no way of correcting the letter. Meanwhile, UT continued to collect the $290.70 premium for insurance. The last collection was May 5, 2023, with the payment processed by UT System UTBB UTBB6001498774. They also processed a payment on April 5, 2023, for $290.70 despite terminating the insurance on March 1, 2023, the date of my cataract surgery. They even processed a $290.70 payment on March 6, 2023, six days after cancelling the insurance. They still have not sent me an official notice of the termination and the reasons for their action.

Summary of complaint:

1. Without notice, warning, or provocation, the insurance I have been paying for years was terminated by some computer program.

2. The reason for the termination is not available or clear and it is not known why the insurance was continued for years while I was healthy as a horse and then stopped when I started to need it because I was sick.

3. If I am not covered by insurance, it is not fair or reasonable for the company to still collect the premiums.

Requested relief:

Get them to reinstate my insurance.

I have a feeling the algorithmic program used against us is used against many old people to maximize insurance company profits. We need your help to defend us from this abuse and discrimination on the basis of age and illness.

The senator knew all the tricks:

<u>Slow pay, the low pay, the no pay.</u>

He knew about denials and refusal to pay because of "experimental" or "not necessary." He knew the cancellation was not unusual when the patient is in the older age group. However, he told me a specific provision of the Affordable Care Act forbids using a computer program to terminate insurance. I used that provision, with the help of Senator Richard Blumenthal's countervailing power to get the insurance reinstated.

I also complained to the Federal Trade Commission, who accepted my complaint and put it on their website. And I complained to the Civil Rights Commission that I was terminated because of my age and that this termination was a violation of law, as it was based on discrimination because I was old. The Civil Rights judge was sympatico, but after a two-month review, she concluded that there was insufficient evidence that the termination was based on age. The reason for termination was deemed a proprietary secret not available to the judge, so she said she was powerless to help.

The medical societies have been screaming for transparency in dealing with insurance. Now, I know why. It is really difficult to counter an opposing argument if you don't know what the argument is. It is impossible to dispute counter-evidence if you can't examine that evidence. The secrecy has to stop so we can uncover the true reasons for delay and denial. My hunch is that the basis is not medical but fiscal. The aim is to maximize profit by minimizing payment. In my view, insurance is hiding the real reasons to protect their bailiwick.

I also filed complaints with Ray Scott, the benefit manager for University of Texas retirees, and I worked with Mary Fox, who works with the Texas Medical Association to help doctors collect from insurance companies. I filed appeals with BCBS. All of that got nowhere. After many letters and telephone calls, Blue Cross and Blue Shield agreed that they had approved the cataract surgery (that fact was a matter of record). But they maintain that approval and preauthorization have nothing whatever to do with whether they would pay or not. "Approvals and payment are separate issues," said my health representative (really a BCBS employee). She said they would pay what was due under the policy, and that was $12. And yes, they did pay a whole $12 of the over $5,000 bill for surgery and the $2,500 Surgi Center bill. My health representative said the remaining $7,488 part of the bill was now my obligation and not theirs.

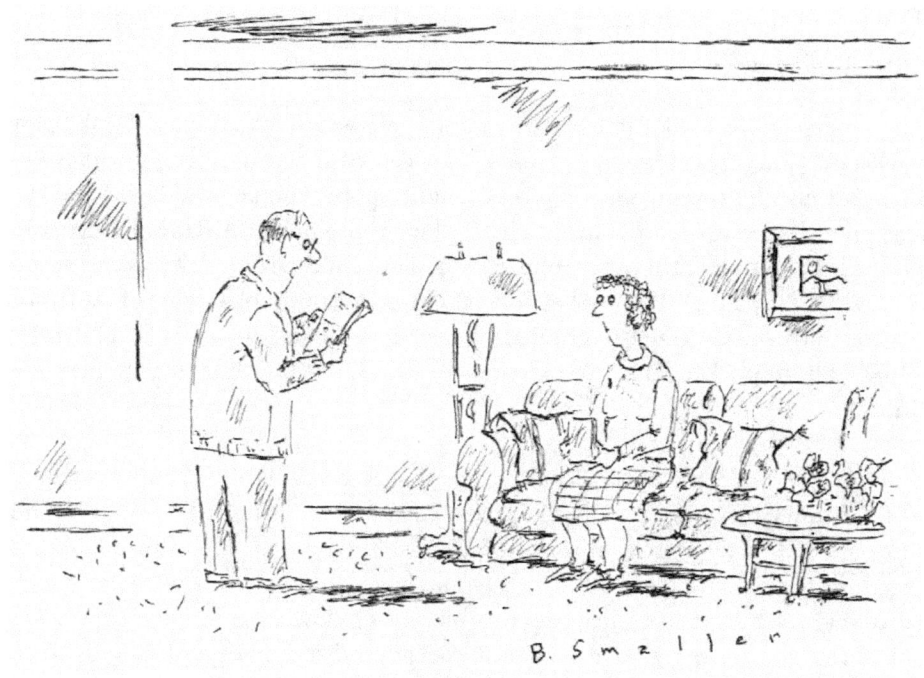

"It says, 'This enormous medical bill is being sent to you on the off chance that you might go ahead and pay it.'"

Whew! I was a slow learner when it came to my own insurance situation. I should have signed up for Medicare Part B when I was 65. I was eligible because I had paid into the system for decades. But the stated benefits on the UT Select Website looked better, so I enrolled in the program for spouses of University of Texas employees. I was eligible for UT Select because for decades, my wife Ethel ran the blood bank at University of Texas Medical Branch.

Don't learn the hard way, the way I did.

My advice:

<u>Enroll when you are eligible in traditional Medicare A and B (not Medicare Advantage). Avoid, if possible, insurance schemes that are in any way connected with private profit.</u>

Don't be fooled by the hype, the way I was. I was fooled by the sales-type documents provided on the website by UT Select and the agent for UT Select, BCBS.

The documents were the come-on that tended to make everything look as rosy and as good as possible.

After much more work, and my threatening a lawsuit, BCBS paid $1,000 for the cataract surgery. Merciful Doctor Chu accepted that as her fee. The anesthesiologists also let me off out of professional respect. The anesthesia for the eye lens procedure was $1,566 plus $128.19, the "ANESTHESIA RISK-RELATED QUALIFIER AGE." Thus, the total anesthesia bill was $1,694. BCBS Insurance paid $25.64. I paid $102.55. They let me off for $1,566, probably from the kindness of Billy, the Certified Registered Nurse Anesthetist. I paid the Surgi Center $1,661 out of pocket. The Surgi Center fee was $2,500, so they too let me off a little.

The irony of this Kafkaesque situation was that Rebecca, the woman who schedules Doctor Chu's surgery, advised me to consider not using the insurance and just paying directly myself. She quoted $1,900 for the right eye. Thus, being insured led to a much bigger bill than I would have had to pay if I were just a cash customer. Cash customers help doctors by cutting down the massive paperwork and stupid insurance rigamarole that physicians and staff have to deal with when insurance is involved. My dermatologist routinely gives me a 30% discount if I pay cash and don't use insurance. Under those conditions, my bill for a visit is usually a very reasonable $36.

MODERN ENCOUNTER FOUR

MISDIAGNOSIS IN THE EMERGENCY ROOM AND SUBSEQUENT ADMISSION TO THE INTENSIVE CARE UNIT

MODERN ENCOUNTER FOUR: MISDIAGNOSIS IN THE EMERGENCY ROOM AND SUBSEQUENT ADMISSION TO THE INTENSIVE CARE UNIT

◆ ◆ ◆

June 24, 2023, I developed fever and rigors (rigors—shaking chills).

In the emergency room of Methodist Hospital, a chest x-ray was done, an electrocardiogram, an abdominal ultrasound, a complete blood count, and a urinalysis. The white blood count was elevated with a shift to the type of white blood cells seen in bacterial infection. And I had rigors, the shaking chills characteristic of a bacterial infection. All the tests for viral infection, including blood tests for COVID, influenza A & B, and respiratory syncytial virus, were negative. Nevertheless, I was diagnosed as having a viral illness of unknown type and sent home. Two days later, June 26, 2023, I became so weak I was unable to get out of the bathtub. Ethel called 911, and men lifted me naked into the ambulance, which transported me back to Houston Methodist, where I was admitted to the intensive care unit and treated for sepsis after four blood cultures returned positive for bacteria. Therefore, in my view, the diagnosis of virus illness was wrong from the start and proven wrong by the subsequent correct diagnosis. In my view, this emergency room visit care was very poor and probably approached gross malpractice on the part of the emergency room doctors.

Interestingly, Houston Methodist Hospital disclaims any responsibility. Their letter, June 20, 2024, says: "Houston Methodist does not employ physicians in the emergency department, but rather they are independent contractors. Any additional concerns regarding your care can be addressed to US Acute Care Solutions at 1-855-687-0618."

My answer to that was: "But the bill came from Houston Methodist and not from any doctor or from US Acute Care."

No answer to that.

"Furthermore, the code for the emergency room visit was Class V—severe life-threatening illness, and yet I was discharged home. Kind of a contradiction here, don't you think? Severe life-threatening illness for billing purposes, but sent home with diagnosis of a (trivial) viral illness."

No answer to that either.

Big institutions like Houston Methodist Hospital are very reluctant to admit a mistake. It would be very rare for the ordinary patient to get an apology or a reduction in the bill, even when obvious mistakes had been made.

About the Quality of Care

Four board-certified physicians have reviewed the situation at my request. They all agree that the diagnosis of viral illness was wrong, and they all consider this "gross malpractice"(1) or "outrageous malpractice"(3). The standard of care should have been:

1. Admit the patient

2. Draw blood cultures

3. Immediately start antibiotic treatments

If the standard of care had been followed instead of ordering a bunch of very expensive tests that showed little, then I would have been saved lots of pain, trouble, and expense.

Not only was the care outrageous, but so were the bills –

Ambulance Bill

City of Nassau Bay Ambulance Service—$1,652.40, of which BCBS paid $180.50, and I got stuck with $1,471.80. Ugh! Low pay again. My fear is they are doing this to normal people (not like me, who is not normal and never was normal) who'n't have the energy or the time or the money to oppose them. Some victims are probably too sick, too stupid, or too dead to do anything. Of course, I filed an appeal with BCBS, playing the claims game. That appeal was rejected because "BCBS determines the value of the service and pays accordingly." Note that their explanation of why they did not pay is merely a restatement that they are not paying. They are not giving a real reason. So, I appealed again. This time, the appeal went to an independent doctor who agreed BCBS should have paid more for ambulance service and approved my appeal. Hooray! I got a notice that, subject to review by BCBS, I might get an additional $749.50. The notice seemed to say BCBS reserved the right to overrule the independent reviewer's decision on the appeal and determine in their sole discretion whether they should pay more or not. But (by mistake?) the $749.50 was sent by BCBS to the ambulance billing service, and they said they sent me a check on 10/14/2024 for $749.50, which I didn't receive. Because I did not get the check, the question devolved into whether it was sent and lost in the mail, or deposited by the wrong person, or they didn't really send it at all. More than a month was spent on the phone trying to get the money I was entitled to, but nothing was happening, so I wrote a nasty letter.

March 7, 2025

City of Nassau Bay

c/o EMS Billing Services

PO Box 747

Wheeling, IL 60090-0747

Once again, I call your attention to your failure to refund $749.50 to me. The second call to you about this matter was made today. I have been on hold for over 30 minutes and I am tired of waiting. To review the situation:

Run Number NBTX-23-679.1 on 06/25/2023 resulted in a bill of $1,471.90 which was paid to you on 9/7/2023 via American Express. On July 24, 2023 Blue Cross and Blue Shield of Texas approved my appeal and paid you an additional $749.50. That amount was never paid to me as it should have been. I am now demanding payment. Please send a check to me at the address above.

If you did send a check and it was cashed, then someone other than myself has stolen the money. Find out who that was and act accordingly.

If I don't receive the refund from you by March 30, I shall file a lawsuit against you and the city of Nassau Bay for the amount due plus interest and punitive damages for this gross delay.

Bernard M. Patten, MD. FACP, FRSM, FTNS, FAAN

Dadpatten@aol.com

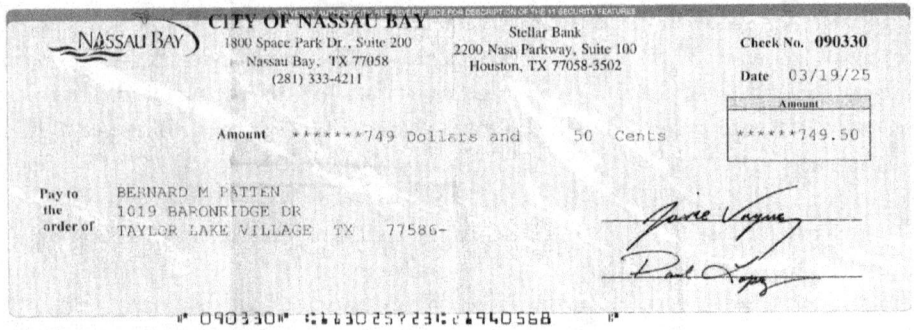

Victory! The check arrived March 19, 2025

Lesson: Never give up. That is what they want you to do. That is a key point in playing the claims game. Do not be fatigued into compliance.

<u>Keep fighting for what you deserve.</u>

Take this knowledge and use it wisely.

Hospital Bills

Medicare Part A paid $21,000 to the Methodist Hospital. Medicare Part A also paid $31,000 to PAM (Post Acute Medicine) South for rehabilitation. But BCBS failed to pay for most of the doctor bills. I appealed again. That got nowhere. So, I hired a lawyer (Jordin Nolan) who will send them a nasty letter and, if that does not work, sue them. Eventually, we will see what judge and jury think of BCBS and how they treated me.

Houston Methodist Emergency Room Bill—$11,609.50

Please do this. Look at the website and discover what the reasonable and average costs for medical things are according to your zip code. **(Texashealthcarecosts.org)**

This will be an eye-opening experience for you, as it was for me. Methodist Hospital is number one, I think, in charges. No question in my mind about it.

Take a look at the bill I got and think about how you would handle it. Remember the basic principle is:

<u>They can bill what they wish, but whether they get paid is a different story.</u>

Also, keep in mind that these numbers on a piece of paper represent money even though you don't see the green. You need to be proactive rather than passive when responding to medical bills.

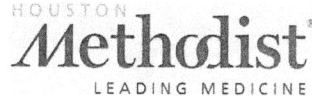

LEADING MEDICINE

PO Box 3133
Houston, TX 77253-3133

05/05/24

Bernard M Md Patten
1019 Baronridge Dr

SEABROOK, TX 77586

Guarantor ID: 2623912

Visit Coverages:

Blue Cross Blue Shield - BCBS Choice PPO

This is an itemization of your medical services for:

Patient:	Patten,Bernard M Md	Admission Date:	06/24/23
Hospital Account:	4502456027	Discharge Date:	06/24/23

Hospital Charges

Date	Rev Code	Procedure Code	Description	Qty	Amount
06/24/23	0324	32400001	HC Chest 2 Views	1	1,312.00
06/24/23	0250	J7030	Sodium Chloride 0.9 % Solution (0338-0049-04)	1	250.50
06/24/23	0402	40200006	HC US Abdominal Limited	1	2,727.00
06/24/23	0450	45000005	HC ER Visit Level V	1	4,222.00
06/24/23	0310	31000321	HC Sars-Cov-2 /Influenza/Rsv	1	445.00
06/24/23	0307	30700002	HC Urinalysis Chemical & Micro	1	408.00
06/24/23	0301	30100005	HC Comprehensive Metabolic Panel	1	884.00
06/24/23	0305	30500006	HC Complete Bld Count W/Auto Diff	1	266.00
06/24/23	0730	73000001	HC Electrocardiogram	1	1,095.00
			Total Charges		11,609.50

Hospital Payments and Adjustments

Date	Description	Amount
	Blue Cross Blue Shield Payments and Adjustments	-5,977.50

Current Hospital Account Balance: 5,632.00
Current Professional Services Balance: 0.00

THE GREAT AMERICAN MEDICAL SHOW

Here's another bill to practice on. Study it carefully and write your analysis. After you have written your reply, read my letter. Some items are not on the surface of the bill, and I had to do work to find the previous paid checks, and I had to look at the alleged provider's (Tiffany Queeney's) website.

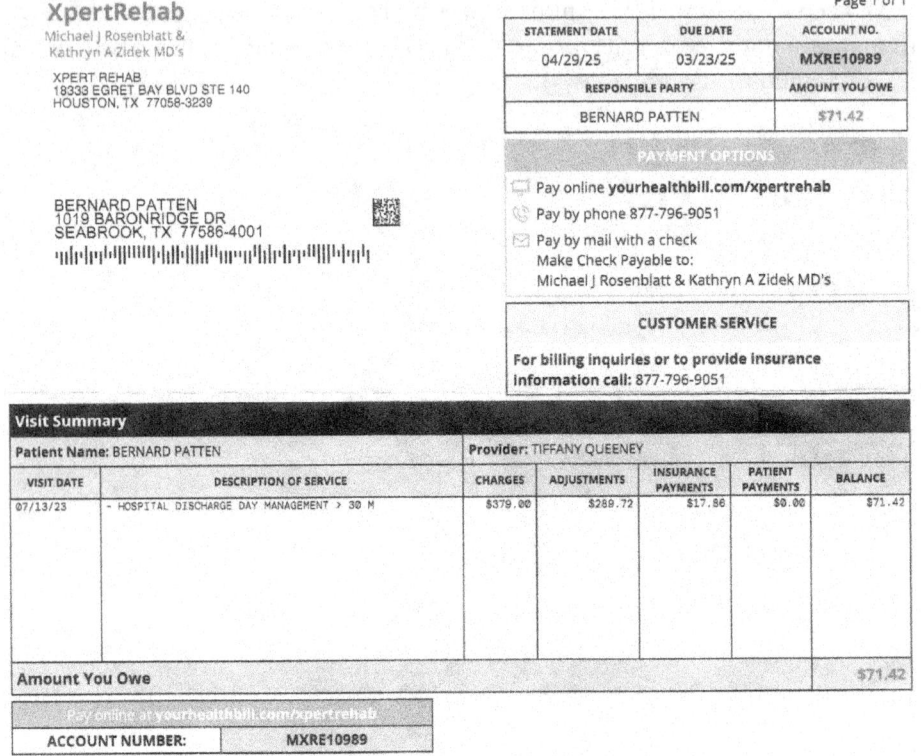

May 10, 2025

Holy cow! Another bill from you all. I already paid Michael Rosenblatt $1,006.17 on 9/4/2024 with check 2740, and also paid again on 2/25/2024 with check 2725. When will you stop billing? When is enough, enough?

Please answer the following by the end of May:

What service was actually done by Queeny on 7/13/23? Send me the written record proof of service. Neither I nor my wife remembers her.

Why was the bill sent so late? Almost two years later?

Why is this not a surprise bill? It certainly surprised me.

Why is the check in payment to go to Rosenblatt when the supposed service was done by Queeney?

Why is the due date 3/23/25 actually before the billing date of 4/29/25? Are we overdue even before we get a bill? This shows how careless you are in billing.

Why does Queeney's website say she accepts assignments and insurance as full payment, and yet she still bills me for more money?

Many thanks for a fast reply. Do not ignore this letter.

Bernard M. Patten, MD. FACP, FRSM, FTNS, FAAN

Reply received May 16, 2025, 12:57 PM via voice mail:

"Hi, Dr. Patten, this is Jill calling from Dr. Rosenblatt. I'm calling to let you know we show zero balance on your account. So, please disregard whatever statement that you received. We was (sic) having some technical issues with our billing statement company. So, please disregard the account as a zero balance. Zero balance. Thank you."

Lesson: Oh well, nothing is perfect in this wide world. Jill might benefit from some instruction in proper usage and clear expression. But the meaning comes through. She is saying: **Forget the bill**.

My heart goes out to most people who would receive a bill like this and just (reluctantly) pay it. Notice the first item I asked for was the written proof of service. After almost two years, they would have to spend considerable time and energy in trying to find such a record if in fact it still existed or if it ever existed. My take on this bill is that the service did not take place, and this is a bill for work not done. My statement that they should not ignore the letter probably scared them, and they realized discretion was the better part of valor.

My general approach is to inspect the bill for what every Irishman wants—talking points. Medical billing in general is a mess. You will not have trouble finding problems in most medical bills and those problems will work in your favor if you know how to use them.

<u>Look for double-billing, excessive coding, services not rendered, math errors, wrong dates of service, and delayed and surprise billing.</u>

Look at the date of the Methodist ER bill. The date is May 5, 2024, for service on June 24, 2023. Why the long delay in billing? If you ask Methodist Guest Relations, they will tell you they don't know. That is an unsatisfactory answer and a reason to claim the bill is a "Surprise Bill." In a sense, this is a surprise bill: It surprised me because it came many moons after the service, and it is for a medical service that made major errors in diagnosis and treatment. I sent Methodist a letter politely claiming this is a surprise bill and, therefore, not legal. With my letter, I enclosed a seven-page booklet by Texas Health Resources explaining my rights.

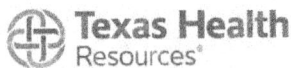

Q
SEARCH

☏
1-877-847-9355

☰
MORE

Costs & Billing

Federal Surprise Billing Act

Helpful information about balance billing

Your Rights and Protections against Surprise Medical Bills

Spanish | Arabic | Vietnamese | French | Burmese
Korean | Farsi | Chinese | Nepali | Mandarin | Hindi
Amharic | Swahili | Portuguese | Urdu | Japanese
Laotian

When you get emergency care or get treated by an out-of-network provider at an in-network hospital or ambulatory surgical center, you are protected from balance billing. In these cases, you shouldn't be charged more than your plan's copayments, coinsurance and/or deductible. See Frequently Asked Questions and Answers for more information.

What is "balance billing" (sometimes called "surprise billing")?

When you see a doctor or other health care provider, you may owe certain out-of-pocket costs, such as a

Glancing over this booklet, I see the law is quite complex and even convoluted. Doubtful that even a trained lawyer will understand it. All that uncertainty works to your advantage and will instill the fear of the law into the corporate giant that is behind this bill. It is for sure that none of the doctors who worked on my case have any idea of how much is being billed for their services. The bill is coming from the administration, probably corporate administration, whose main attention is focused on money. The bill is not from the medical personnel. The doctors are out of the billing loop for sure because the doctors themselves would consider the bill outrageous. How do I know? I asked them. They have no control over how much is billed or when the bills are sent out. Quote: "We know nothing."

Next, the charges are sky high and out of line with anything remotely reasonable. The amount they say I owe—$5,632—stuns me. Eleven thousand dollars for a two-hour visit to the ER! The bill is outrageous, even though BCBS paid $5,977.50.

Suggested Approach To Outrageous Bills

You can't just claim it is outrageous. You have to have backup. That's where the opinions of my physician friends came in, and that is where the Texas website about the usual charges helps support your argument. If you don't have physician friends, get busy and make them.

In another letter to Methodist, I cite some examples:

> "The average cost for a chest X-ray in Houston is $107. Michelle Luschen (board-certified radiologist) says your charge of $1,312 for code 32400001 standard plain film is 'crazy.' All previous chest X-rays on me at Houston Methodist Clear Lake have been billed at $58. The charges for urinalysis, metabolic panel, and CBC exceed the state average costs by over a thousand percent! Nationwide, the charge for an EKG with interpretation is $52 and not Methodist's $1,095, which is 2,105% above the usual fee!"

I should have added, $250 for a normal saline infusion! Who is kidding who? Today on Amazon (January 31, 2025) that amount of normal saline is for sale at $10.78, not the $250 charged by Methodist Hospital.

My letter continues:

"The more I investigate, the worse Methodist Hospital looks. The charges are way out of line with community standards and the standards of the Texas Insurance Board. I review these averages and nationally above, and compare them to the actual charges made by Houston Methodist. Texas standards and the national standards for costs of tests can be checked on the Texas website (**Texashealthcarecosts.org**)."

"In my view, the care was poor in the extreme. Think of this: The billing is for an emergency code, yet I was sent home and emergency care was not given."

As an assistant physician at the New York Hospital Cornell Medical Center (July 1966 to June 1967), I treated 17 patients with sepsis. All the patients were admitted to the hospital because, in the good old days, we did not send patients with sepsis home from the emergency room.

The unofficial protocol, which we all followed, was admission to a regular hospital bed and not to the intensive care unit (ICU). ICU is a terrible experience for any patient with all the noise and lights, and multiple interruptions of rest and sleep. ICU was not needed in the routine care of the usual case of sepsis. Once the patient was in bed, I immediately drew the blood cultures and started antibiotic treatment (known as blast-a-bug). This was done even before doing the history or physical exam because the clinical diagnosis is obvious if you see rigors (the medical term for shivering attacks) and fever in the elderly. My usual Rx for suspected sepsis was 20 million units of penicillin plus methicillin (to cover possible penicillin-resistant bacteria) plus colistin for the gram-negative bacteria. If the patient was immunosuppressed, I would add amphotericin B for suspected fungal sepsis. All that was given intravenously was within the first hour of admission.

The next day, the patient was much better because Blast-a-Bug had killed whatever bug was causing the sepsis. Two days later, the blood cultures would return with sensitivities, and the antibiotic treatment would be adjusted. That was the good old days—fast, effective, usually inexpensive, and certainly dirt cheap when compared to contemporary charges.

Mental Anguish and Unnecessary Pain and Suffering

Imagine how I felt in the hospital ICU, knowing I had sepsis and yet being told, "No treatment until we have a definite diagnosis."

The delay was endangering my life, but I was like most patients in the hospital, unable to do anything about it. Imagine how I felt, knowing what I knew and suffering greatly as my heart, liver, kidneys, and lungs were falling apart.

Then came the most unkindest cut of all. Four blood cultures returned positive for Klebsiella bacteria, establishing a definite diagnosis of sepsis. "We can't start treatment until the sensitivities come back." In other words, more delay, no antibiotic treatment until another lab report comes in. More delay and, in my view, completely unnecessary and dangerous because my vital organs were falling apart. In the old days, we (that is, all doctors at the Cornell Medical Center) would simply make an educated guess about what antibiotic would kill the Klebsiella that was trying to kill me. In a community-acquired infection in a previously healthy person, the bug is usually killed by almost any antibiotic.

Finally, in my case, the sensitivities were reported. They showed, as predicted, that my Klebsiella was sensitive to all the antibiotics (over 27) tested, except ampicillin, to which the bug was partly resistant. But there is a complication: The infectious disease doctor on my case checked with BCBS and found out that the more effective intravenous antibiotic for my sepsis will not be paid for. Hence, she will use the less expensive oral antibiotic. Unbelievable, but true. My wife coughed up the additional $531 for the antibiotic in the hospital, and to be continued during outpatient care. This sounds like the step-up insurance scheme was trying to save money by delaying a more effective treatment, and it probably was. I shudder to think of what might have happened if we went along with the step-up. I might not be here to write my analyses and views. Think about this: what do people do who don't have the money to pay for the more effective treatment? That is wrong, dead wrong. But the dead can't talk about it or complain because they are (you guessed it) dead. It is rather we, the living, who must here highly resolve to vigorously complain and right these wrongs.

In my view, Methodist looks money hungry and seems to be exploiting the public. Methodist must need lots of money to pay for the massive advertising program that features billboards telling the public how great Methodist is. Notice the headline on the ER bill: Methodist LEADING MEDICINE. In my view, self-serving self-praise stinks. The fee for ads in Bloomberg Business Magazine alone must add up to quite a bit of money that, in my opinion, should be better spent on medical care or medical research. Suddenly, I realize the good old days are gone. Medicine has changed. In my day, physicians had a calling that catered to the public health and welfare. Our prime consideration was the patient.

<u>Now, medicine is a business—a big business. It is often impersonally practiced as a faceless corporation, with the focus mainly on bottom-line profits, not the well-being of humanity.</u>

Like big businesses, they advertise. Deep down, I resent that. I think hospitals and physicians who advertise are low-down and dirty and not professional in the old sense that I understood the word *professional*. The ads are usually self-serving and extremely superficial. "Their Orthopedic expertise keeps me moving." "Methodist is number one in Neurological Care in Texas." "Thanks to Methodist for my prostate cancer care, my wife and I are back dancing." "Methodist—Best emergency care in League City."

The ads don't mention that the care for multiple sclerosis, Alzheimer's disease, many kinds of stroke, and many cancers is just a notch above the placebo effect. The ads don't mention that local neurologists think Memorial Hermann Hospital does better on stroke care. The ads don't mention that M.D. Andersen Hospital in Houston, not Methodist, is considered the best cancer hospital in America. Other hospitals are more reasonable with their ads, just a simple alert to the public about what is available: "UTMB—Women's Care," Another bulletin board on Highway 45: "UTMB—Orthopedic Care," and "UTMB knows pediatrics."

When patients judge Methodist, it does look good compared to local hospitals. Methodist gets 4/5 stars; HCA gets 2/5 stars; St. Luke's gets 3/5 stars; and Houston Physicians gets 5/5 stars.

The process of care results for sepsis, the diagnosis that was missed in my visit to the ER, gives Methodist a 74% for treatment of 129 patients, meaning there is need for much improvement. This data is from Medicare results, which you can check online. If you check that website, you will find Methodist does more extensive and more expensive testing than average and charges more. Most of the high-powered expensive tests show no clinically important result, suggesting but not proving the tests should not have been ordered in the first place. Methodist is leading medicine, no question about it, leading in charges.

Methodist is basically a good hospital and the care is above average, but there is room for improvement and that improvement should probably start with a change in administration and management focus and especially a change in attitude.

Result: After six letters back and forth about my ER visit, Methodist offered a 20% discount, which I rejected. I told them for me to pay anything would be a tacit admission or a condolence of the care and that is not my view or position. So, they cancelled the entire $5,632 current hospital account balance and I ended up paying nothing for that emergency room catastrophe.

Practice working out on the following bill. See if you can spot the problems and talking points. Write down your analysis so you don't fool yourself into thinking you did a better job at analysis than you did. After you finished, take a look at my discussion. There are several points about this bill under the surface that I know are defective. I will tell you about them when you finish your work and analysis.

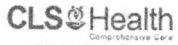

CLS Health
Comprehensive Care
PO BOX 58688
Webster, TX 77598
281-694-5972

Statement Date	Invoice Number	Page
01/04/2024	IDCLS PATBE000	1

Guarantor	Due Date	Payment Due
BERNARD M.	Upon Receipt	1,177.00

Pay Online
Go to: cls.health/payment
or scan the QR Code

BERNARD M. PATTEN
1019 BARONRIDGE DR
SEABROOK, TX 77586-4001

Make Checks Payable To:
INFECTIOUS DISEASES CLINIC AT
PO BOX 58688
Webster, TX 77598

Date of Last Payment:	Amount of Last Payment: 0.00	Account Balance $ 1177.00

Patient:	Rendering Physician:	Chart Number:	Place of Service:	Date of Birth:
BERNARD M. PATTEN	MICHELLE ONORATO MD	PATBE000	INFECTIOUS	03/23/1941

Dates	Procedure	Description	Modifier	Charge	Paid By Applied to Patient Deductible	Paid by BLUE	Adjustments	Remainder
07/26/23	99204	OFFICE VIST NEW LEVEL 4		503.00		0.00		503.00

Patient:	Rendering Physician:	Chart Number:	Place of Service:	Date of Birth:
BERNARD M. PATTEN	MICHELLE ONORATO MD	PATBE000	INFECTIOUS	03/23/1941

Dates	Procedure	Description	Modifier	Charge	Paid By Applied to Patient Deductible	Paid by BLUE	Adjustments	Remainder
08/11/23	99212	OFFICE VIST EST LEVEL 2	25	171.00		0.00		171.00

Patient:	Rendering Physician:	Chart Number:	Place of Service:	Date of Birth:
BERNARD M. PATTEN	MICHELLE ONORATO MD	PATBE000	INFECTIOUS	03/23/1941

Dates	Procedure	Description	Modifier	Charge	Paid By Applied to Patient Deductible	Paid by MEDICARE	Adjustments	Remainder
07/26/23	99204	OFFICE VIST NEW LEVEL 4		503.00		0.00		503.00

My office has been trying to reach you via phone with no response. Please contact my office at your earliest convenience to update your account information. If you do not respond in business days, the full balance will be posted to patient responsibility. Have a question about your balance, or need to update your insurance information with us? Call 281-694-5972 To make a payment online, go to cls.health/payment. If remitting payment via mail in check, Please include statement.

Amount Due
1,177.00

Point One: This bill is dated January 4, 2024, for services July 26, 2023, and August 11, 2023. Why the long delay? Did you raise the question of a surprise billing because of the long delay? Did you notice that the office visit on July 26, 2023, is billed twice, once on top of the bill and once on the bottom? Therefore, this bill is double billing for the exact same date with the exact same codes and exact same charge. The charge amount of $503 has also been doubled and added to the total bill, which is $1,177.

Delayed bills bother me because I know that when some people are running low on money, they tell the secretaries to search the files for a billable client. The late bill is sent out in the hope that it might be paid. My mother-in-law worked for a lawyer and told me that is exactly what they did when they were low on cash.

Further information: The rest of this bill is defective because the visit on July 26, 2023, is coded as a new patient visit when I was not new. That's overbilling because the usually acceptable fee for a new patient is larger than the fee for a patient who is already in the system. New patients require more work than patients already known to the doctor and staff. The actual visit lasted only ten minutes. I was not examined. Michelle just asked how I was doing and made a few remarks about how lucky I was to survive. At most, this visit was a level 2 and not a level 4. My wife, who is a board-certified internist, was with me at the time. She agrees this was not a level 4, comprehensive complex visit. It was merely routine; therefore, level 2.

Always keep records of your visits and note the time involved. Our wait for that visit was close to an hour. I know doctors are busy, but still, something has to be done about wait time. There is way too much waiting.

Another Point: You don't know about this, but Ethel and I do. The visit on August 11, 2023, never took place. This is a bill for service never rendered. I called and asked the secretary to look up the medical record, which I knew didn't exist because the visit didn't happen. The secretary searched the medical records and found no record of that visit. She admitted there was no record, but thought the bill was for removing the intravenous catheter. The catheter was removed that day by the infusion service nurse. The doctor was nowhere in sight, and yet the doctor billed it as an office visit. We had already paid for the infusion service for the nurse to remove the PIC line. So, there was no legitimate reason to bill us again for the service already paid for. The secretary, bless her heart, agreed.

Result: Because of all the outrageous mistakes, this entire bill for $1,177 was cancelled.

Another example: I received a bill for a little over $3,000 from an organization that calls itself "Expert MDs." To me, that's a red flag. Self-praise stinks. Calling themselves Expert MDs does not make them so and certainly does not prove they are experts. It does tend to make them look like braggarts.

The bill demanded payment to a physician whose name was different from the physician who allegedly performed six complex evaluations on separate days. As usual, the bill was about a year overdue and, therefore, a surprise in the sense that it was unexpected. And, get this, the year of all the alleged services was 1943, when I was two years old and in New York City, not in Texas or in the Methodist Hospital. Obviously, an error, probably a series of typos when someone was sleeping at the switch and not thinking. But still, this is a talking point tending to demonstrate carelessness in billing. My letter was brief:

> "I don't remember the doctor or the service. Send me the medical record that proves the service, and I shall be happy to consider paying."

This is a request that usually works to your advantage for several reasons:

1. The service may not have been performed and probably was over-coded.

    OR:

2. The service was performed, but they don't have a record of it.

    OR:

3. The record is embedded in the 716 pages of hospital notes and will be difficult, if not impossible, to find. Modern records are so thick that no one has time to read them. Everyone puts something in it. The nurses, the doctors, the pharmacist, the social worker, the hospital-appointed reviewer, the intern, the resident, the clinical psychologist, and even the business office.

Result: Several months have gone by, and there have been no more demands for payment from Expert MDs. Result: Questioning the bill and asking for evidence got me out of paying over $3,000.

It damages my mental health to think too much about my stay in the intensive care unit. Each time I bring an image to mind, I get a flashback back and last night, there was the usual trouble with my sleep. Instead of giving a detailed narration, I wish to point out some personal observations which may be helpful to you. This will be done by topic.

Observations That May Be Helpful to You

Intensive Care Unit: My experience there was horrible and has caused post-traumatic stress disorder. There is too much light and too much noise, and too many machines attached to me. Are they all necessary? Often, often too often, the alarms go off and nurses rush in to find that an electrode was misplaced, and I am still alive. Meanwhile, my blood pressure and anxiety level have jumped sky high. Why can't the monitoring be done remotely at the nurses' station so that the patient may rest?

Oh yeah, about rest—forget it. Rest is almost impossible. As soon as I doze off, someone comes to take a chest X-ray or a blood test or to check my oxygen or to give me medicine or to take my blood pressure and pulse rate (even though they are clearly displayed on the overhead monitor) or to see if I am still alive.

ICU = no real rest for the sick or weary.

Rest, according to the Journal of the American Medical Association (JAMA. 1925:84(5):371), is very important and a major discovery of the Trudeau Sanatorium, 1885-1925, built before hospitals became machines for healing and when fields and gardens surrounded Queens Village, my childhood home. "Above all, there was an emphasis on the importance of rest." The JAMA article lauds rest as a fundamental principle of medical treatment. Anyone who has been sick knows how important rest is to aid recovery. Often, the only thing the sick person needs is adequate rest. In fact, sometimes rest is all a sick person can do.

Here's my point:

Rest is important in helping the patient defeat the disease.

Therefore, ICU violates one of the most ancient and most important, and most respected fundamental principles of medicine—REST.

Hippocrates, the father of medicine, was famously said to have enjoined his followers: "First, do no harm." Ho ho ho. It is highly unlikely he said such. It does not appear in any of Hippocrates' writings. The correct quote is "Practice two things in your dealing with disease: either help or do not harm the patient." Makes sense.

The real statement was changed by Thomas Inman, a British surgeon, whose other claim to fame was, well, nothing. In my view, Hippocrates' major discovery, for which he deserves a Nobel Prize, was that diseases are caused by **nature** and not by **actions of the gods**, as had previously been believed. Toning down the super- natural in medical care was a great advance in human thinking.

Anyway, the do no harm principle has become a sacred motto of the medical profession and will be the same for all eternity. ICU violates that principle, and measures should be taken to make it a patient-friendly place. Also, we need a prospective scientific clinical study to compare the results of sepsis care in two matched groups of patients, half treated in the ICU and half treated on the usual hospital floor, as I discussed was the standard of care at the New York Hospital when I was a house officer. Maybe there is too much ICU in the same way that there was in the old days too much bed rest for patients with heart attacks, or too much bleeding, or too many mercury enemas, or too much radon inhalation. The conjecture that ICU is better has never been proven and needs to be objectively addressed.

Another complaint about the ICU was that as a patient, I am treated like a baby, virtually helpless and not in control. The hospital and the staff are in complete control. They don't even give me an illusion of being in control or having much of a say-so. Doctors are chosen not by me but by the team. No one asked if I was OK with any of the 17 medicines I was taking. No one explained why I needed a chest X-ray every day and a complete blood count and metabolic screen every day. I felt isolated and alone. The reason I felt that way was that I was isolated and alone.

Food: Surprisingly good. Usually served on time and properly cooked. The food looked good, smelled good, and tasted good. This was a big plus and totally un- expected.

Physical therapy (PT) and occupational therapy (OT): Two activities looked down on by the team, but specifically requested by me. Both are wonderful. PT came and got me out of bed and walking with a stroller. When I got tired, I rested. After recovering, we went to work again. Every day saw progress and convinced me I was on the road to Wellville.

A positive mental attitude helps any patient recover.

OT got me out of bed and onto the bedside chair. This made a gigantic differ- ence in my outlook. Then OT got me a bedside commode. This was a wonderful relief from the tedium of the bedpan. I was being potty-trained all over again.

OT taught me how to manage trailing urine bags, intravenous drip stands, and two liver tubes draining pus. And merciful OT, taught me how to shower while protecting what needed protection. Kudos and three cheers for PT and OT. But why, oh why, did I never get a bill from them? I would have paid right away. The same thing happened with the neurologist whom I loved and who helped run my case effectively. She never billed me. I figured she wouldn't bill me. And she didn't bill insurance. She performed too much like a professional from the bygone era. She wasn't part of the team, and she went out of her way to set the team straight on multiple issues. Thank God!

Doctors: Ugh! I regret having to give my firm and truthful appraisal. If I don't, how will you and the public know the difference. I did a poor job of selecting my doctors in the ICU because I didn't select them. They were forced on me for better or worse by the hospital.

Most of the doctors seemed overworked and tired. They rarely addressed me directly. They should always be seated when talking to patients. Nope, not them. They should never appear to be in a hurry. Nope, not them. They are so green, they don't even know where to place the stethoscope to properly listen to heart valves. I'm in a state of shock. The rest of the physical exams, with two exceptions, were worthless and probably done just to have something on record that might indicate they actually did an exam. In case I died, they could prove to the lawyers in a malpractice case that they examined me. That's all their fast, lousy exam accomplishes.

The neurologist was an absolute gem. She did a detailed exam and proved I had a combined system's disease due to B12 deficiency. She went out of her way to tell the group that I didn't have DTs (delirium tremens) because I was fully oriented and not delirious. Nevertheless, my team continued Librium on the "outside possibility of DTs." I was beginning to dislike the *team* approach to my case. Obviously, no one on the team had ever seen a patient with DTs. I longed for the good old days when there was one doctor, whom I knew and liked and trusted, who was in charge and who liked me and listened.

When there was a question of what the golf ball-sized lesions in my liver were, the neurologist produced a clinical paper describing a large number of cases of Klebsiella sepsis, where 72% of patients had liver abscesses. That changed the thinking of the team from hopeless cancer metastatic to the liver to pus that needed to be drained. The neurologist actually also changed the thinking of the so-called infectious disease expert who had been assigned my case. Now the infectious disease specialist thought I didn't, perhaps, have metastatic cancer in my liver.

The GI (gastroenterology) guy, Michel, was also wonderful. He agreed with the neurologist about the DTs and the combined systems disease and wrote the same in my chart. "Besides," he wrote about delirium tremens, "He doesn't drink enough to be in withdrawal." Nevertheless, the team continued the Librium on the "outside chance of DTs." Not only had no one on my team ever seen a case of DTs, but even more discouraging was that they were unwilling to follow the expert advice of the neurologist and the gastroenterologist.

And talking about GI, Michel's history and physical examination met and exceeded accepted national standards. He and the neurologist were the only ones who knew my family history, personal history, social history, previous medical problems, and review of systems. He spoke to me on my level, and by his body language and facial expression, I knew he was deeply concerned about my welfare. "What's my prognosis?" I asked. He shook his head. "Hard to say." The reality was, of course, he had no idea of what would happen to me. I knew this, but childishly hoped he would tell me things would be fine.

I am sure Michel would recognize me on the street, and that none of the parade of specialists and none of my team of doctors would either recognize me or know my name. When Michel's bill came, I paid it right away.

The team doctors are from a new and different generation. Obviously, for some of them, English is not their original language. I had trouble understanding them on the rare occasion that they talked to me directly. The usual talk was among themselves with many smiles and laughs, leaving me out in the cold and not in the know. Consider this: once the team assigned a consultant to my case, that doctor came every day, whether they were needed or not.

The main doctor on my case went on vacation without saying goodbye. But he did tell my wife and my daughter, Allegra, that he was leaving on vacation. I never did get to know who took his place. Now, they have stripped me of my command. No one asks me what to do. They tell me what to do, and I submit. Once in a hospital, patients become dehumanized. It is much easier to handle them that way. Anomie results. Modern medicine is past its Best Before date.

In my day, I knew my patients very well, and I covered my patients 24/7 by page and phone and thought nothing special about it. The new generation works far less hours and gets vacations and nights off and weekends off. They are right. Long hours did lead to fatigue and errors in judgment. On the other hand, when the doctors changed shifts, I was subject to needless re-exam and errors. The new doctors want more time off, and that is good for them and probably not so good for the patients.

Are the new doctors as good as my generation? No way! My class at P&S had 125 excellent students. Each position in my medical school class had 32 applicants. We, therefore, were a very select group. Twenty or so could walk on water and the rest were more than acceptable. Two have even won Nobel prizes.

Now there are lots more medical schools selecting students from a pool of acceptable applicants that is shrinking. The intelligent students are being enticed away from medicine by computer science, finance, business, and law where the pay is higher.

My teaching of medical students started in 1969 and continued to 1996. During those three decades, I am sure the intellectual horsepower, basic cultural awareness, logical thinking, scientific knowledge, empathy, or any other desirable character trait in a doctor that you can think of has been in decline. There were a few students who I thought should never have started medicine. Nevertheless, the student in the class with the lowest grade point average graduating from a second-rate medical school or osteopathic school will be called *doctor* and will have MD or DO after their name.

Among the blind purchases people make in life is the purchase of medical care. To help you select the right doctor, I wish to tell you what I look for.

1. I want a physician with integrity. His or her advice should be for my benefit and not for them.

2. Next, I would want to check the doctor's knowledge. What medical school did he/she graduate from? Where was the residency? How about board certification? Did they keep up with journal reading, rounds and conferences, and CME (continuing medical education)?

3. What do colleagues think? I should make careful inquiry as to whom I should consult. Being able to do this is a great benefit of being a physician and having physician friends. What is the experience and track record with my illness?

4. After these questions are answered, I consider personality. Sympathetic? Willing to listen? Good communicator? Are we compatible? Some practitioners have empathy; some don't. I don't think it can be learned. If I am

sick and worried, the person who should be making an adjustment is the doctor who is well and not me, the patient, and not you, the patient.

Back to ICU Categories

Nurses: A spectrum, some good and some not so good. Nurses are overworked. Now that hospitals are profit-oriented, they are hiring fewer nurses, and nursing errors have become more common. Many nurses are just going through the motions. Some don't know much. One nurse held me down during a rigor. She kept yelling, "Calm down! You have to calm down." My reply in a very calm voice: "This is a result of the sepsis. I am calm, completely calm." That went through her like a neutrino: no effect. "Calm down!" she shouted.

On the other hand, one nurse was very kind and shampooed my hair, which was much in need. She, Debbie, was the exception, one of the most gentle and indefatigable nurses I ever saw. She met my gaze straight on, gave me the good eye, and softly caressed my hair after she washed it. That's fine with me. She is taking care of me and cares about what happens. Her lesson for the other nurses: "Try a little tenderness."

Amazingly, the most complete analysis of my case (and the only detailed analysis that I found in my chart) was written by a nurse practitioner. Her literary masterpiece had little or no influence on the team.

The lack of criticism of doctors from most patients makes it all too easy for doctors to be pleased with themselves and have a very high opinion of their work. Patients praise when things go right, but hesitate to comment when they don't. Partial selection of evidence leads to false conclusions. When I got sick, I finally realized how little doctors understand about what their patients are going through.

Clergy: Unwanted. I put down that I am an atheist and didn't want spiritual care. They came anyway, surrounded by devoted doting women. "Please leave me alone," I pleaded. "We want you to be reconfirmed in your beliefs. God wants you back. We are praying for you." My reply: "Stop! I don't want any prayers. I am firm in my beliefs. There is no God. There is no heaven. There is no hell. There is no life after death. Having seen all the death and destruction in my practice every god-damn day, I can't believe an all-merciful, all-powerful God would allow it. To me, illness is not something people deserve. The most unfair thing of all is the suffering of children. I have taken care of kids with malignant brain tumors.

"Why would an all-powerful, all-merciful God allow that to happen?"

No answer from the minister. I understand. He doesn't know. Theologians have never come up with a satisfactory answer. They suggest that evil is our own fault because we have free will. Get it? All the bad things are our own fault and not God's fault. Or, they say God works in mysterious ways. What and why? Another smokescreen to obfuscate the paradox that is theodicy, a gigantic discipline to which one of my music teachers has a whole shelf of erudite books. The let-out is that all wrongs will be corrected in the afterlife. Without the promise of an afterlife, most religions would perish. If our lives continue after death, abortion and assisted suicide can't be viewed as absolute evils. If there is really going to be a heavenly banquet after death, why delay?

Tests: You guessed my opinion.

Way too many tests.

And way too much significance is attached to the results. The cardiologist thought I was having a heart attack, even though I had no chest pain and my EKG was normal. He based his diagnosis on one heart enzyme being slightly elevated. The heart was injured. No question about it. But injured by the sepsis and not a heart attack. This heart doctor, against my will, started an anti-platelet drug as would be given for a heart attack. The result was the radiologist would not drain the liver pus until the anti-platelet drug had worn off. That led to a three-day delay in effective treatment and another three days of suffering for me. The heart doctor, like so many of these new doctors, was treating a lab test and not treating the patient. He had also failed to understand the reason for not giving an antiplatelet drug.

Medical Record: A complete mess. My short admission led to 716 pages of mess. The same test results are reported multiple times. There is a lot of cut and paste to bulk up the chart and make it look like a lot more was being done than was being done. Because of the gigantic volume of copied and repeated results, it is very difficult to get any significant information from the chart. When I was in practice, the admission note was about one page, and the discharge summary was maybe two to four pages with a fairly complete report of what was done and why. The discharge summary was dictated, and there was no copy and paste. When I was a sub-intern at Bellview Hospital, where patients were very sick, we were never allowed to write an admission note longer than two paragraphs. When I was a resident at the Neurological Institute of New York, the rule was that all admission notes were limited to one page and one page only.

By now, you know the ritual, and by now, you are tired of hearing the rants about hospitals, doctors, nurses, tests, insurance delays and denials, and you are tired of hearing about overbilling, overcoding, billing for services not done, and so forth. It can be boring dealing with medical problems. But you have to do it just the way you have to do your income tax. Get in the right attitude that every medical bill is usually in some way defective and might be corrected to be lower. Every medical bill is an opportunity to save yourself money. Save money by being an intelligent consumer of medical care and an intelligent payer.

How to Handle Medical Bills

Keep in mind that medical bills are a different breed of cat. The usual cause of a medical debt is an unforeseen illness or a serious accident resulting in hospitalization. Therefore, medical debt is treated with more sympathy than other debt. The medical bill receives special treatment by the credit companies and the law. Credit companies will temporarily disregard any medical bill under $500 or any bill that is less than a year old. The law regards medical debt as non-priority and unsecured in Chapter 7 bankruptcy. Other creditors get the assets first, and often nothing is left to pay the medical debt, which is then discharged. Some medical debts are sold at a fraction (usually $1 per $100) to collection agents. It is then possible for you to purchase the debt and get forgiven for a song. Check this out with non-profit organizations like RIP Medical (now renamed Undue Medical Debt) in Long Island City. That organization has purchased and cancelled over $14.8 billion of medical debt.

<u>Legal handling of medical debt varies in differ states and jurisdictions.</u>

I talked to the local judge of Harris County Precinct 2 about medical debt. He told me he never accepts a suit from a doctor or from a hospital to collect a medical debt. That is the best way of handling it. He hates having to do evictions, but considers many of the evictions reasonable if the renter hasn't paid rent for a long time. For this judge of the peace, medical debt is not a legally enforceable debt.

By the way, if a doctor or a corporation sues you for a medical debt in some other jurisdiction, do not just put the legal papers in a desk drawer and forget about them. You must answer the lawsuit in 30 days, or a default judgment might be issued against you. That could result in the sheriff seizing some of your assets, like your computer or TV, or your Siamese cat. Your written answer should deny everything they accuse you of and should add counterclaims such as malpractice, over-coding, surprise billing, and so forth. You just need to file your answer on time, and usually the case against you will, after a while, be discharged because of non-pursuit by the plaintiff.

The last time I checked, American medical debt amounted to between $200 and $220 billion. That is probably an underestimate because some foolish people convert their medical debt to credit card debt. Don't do that unless you're trying to commit financial suicide. Credit card debt charges sky-high interest and doesn't have the special considerations that medical debt does.

In fact, in America, medical debt is the most common cause of personal bankruptcy, something you should avoid if possible.

Many hospitals are required to offer financial services and charity when patients can't pay. They set up their own criteria on who and what qualifies. In most cases, this will be a frustrating waste of time, and you will feel like hanging yourself. The paperwork will be enormous, and the usual decision will be that you do not qualify.

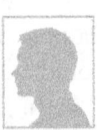

POST-CATARACT LASER SURGERY

MODERN ENCOUNTER FIVE: POST-CATARACT LASER SURGERY

◆ ◆ ◆

Jim was right. The right eye got dim again because the posterior capsule started to scar. The treatment was to burn holes in the tissue to let light in so I could see clearly again. The result was excellent, and so was the experience. This took place in the same Surgi Center with the same eye surgeon, Dr. Kai Chu. But now I no longer had BCBS. Now I was under the kind administrations of Medicare Part A and Part B.

The total bill was $7,877 plus $121.39 for anesthesia.

The encounter was very different. There was no hassle at the check-in desk and very little wait. No one seemed worried about whether Medicare would pay or not. In fact, the contrary was true. They had no doubt they would be paid. Everyone was all smiles about my new insurance coverage. Me too! And here's the miracle: Of the total bill of $7,877, my obligation was $60.38 plus $77.87 for anesthesia, all of which I happily paid with my American Express credit card.

Senator Bernie Sanders has the right idea about Medicare for all. In my view, it would save lots of time and money by removing the profit motives from the loop.

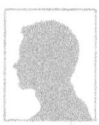

POSSIBLE CANCER OF THE SKIN

MODERN ENCOUNTER SIX: POSSIBLE CANCER OF THE SKIN

◆ ◆ ◆

Recently, I hit my leg on an open draw and developed a large white lesion at the injury site. Donna Sue Dolle, my primary care doctor, said she didn't like the way it looked and thought it was cancer. Another physician, board-certified in Internal Medicine, said the same, so I called my dermatologist for an appointment. Because I was an established patient, the wait time for an appointment was only two months. The idea of waiting that long for a skin cancer didn't bother me because the lesion was in an area of the leg that I could reach and easily do a surgical removal if needed. Besides, my daughter, Allegra (also an MD), looked at the photos and said the lesion was a keratoma. She said this is a syndrome in old men: They hit the anterior part of their leg, and the skin goes into overdrive, producing a keratoma that looks like a cancer but is benign and will disappear by itself.

It pays to have a doctor in the family. Allegra was right. By the time the two months were up, the supposed skin cancer had disappeared.

I kept the Derm appointment anyway. The appointment was for 8:30, and I arrived at 8. I had decided in advance that I would not wait more than an hour past my appointment time. At 9:30, I will leave. Meanwhile, I read an excellent book, Lewis Thomas's *The Lives of a Cell*. Always bring something to your medical visit to help you get through the wait time.

At 9:29, with only one minute to go, I got up to tell the admission clerk I was leaving, but at that very moment, the nurse called me in. The nurse talked to me about why I was there and then told me to undress for a skin check. "The doctor will be in soon."

Again, the "soon" was a medical soon. When the doctor arrived, I waited in the cold room dressed only in my underpants for about 22 minutes. She apologized for the delay but she did not say why she was late. She inspected my leg with a magnifier and agreed that nothing was there, and she thought the problem was a keratoma due to trauma that had cured itself. She wrote the diagnosis on a paper and gave it to me so I could look it up on the internet. Then, I showed her the picture of what had been on my leg, the supposed cancer. Janice looked it over carefully and shook her head. "It does look like a cancer. If I had seen this, I would have called you in for a biopsy."

In my view, most of this is unacceptable: the two-month wait to actually see the doctor and the long wait in the waiting room beyond the appointment time. But the long wait to get to the dermatologist did save me the trouble of getting a biopsy, the costs of surgery, the cost of follow-up examination, and the cost of a report by the pathologist. Also saved was the worry about biopsy results and the risk of surgical infection, as there was no surgery. Natural healing worked its miracle.

<u>Often, no treatment is the best treatment.</u>

According to the AARP Bulletin January/February 2025, page 7, the average wait for new patients to see a physician is 26 days. In a medical emergency, the situation can become even more frightening: Twenty-two percent of acutely ill patients 65 or older had to wait six days or more for an appointment, according to a 2021 survey by the Commonwealth Fund. This is a crisis that's getting worse rapidly. Maybe telemedicine will cut the travel and wait times. That's my hope.

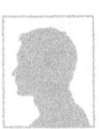

ENCOUNTER THE LAST

ENCOUNTER THE LAST

◆ ◆ ◆

On September 4, 2024, Ethel needed the battery of her pacemaker replaced. We had an appointment at the University of Texas Medical Branch at noon to check in. We arrived early at 11:30 because there was little traffic on the way, and the hospital parking was a breeze. The parking was primarily for the convenience of patients, so we had no problem parking close to the hospital entrance. Someone had done serious thinking about patient comfort and convenience. Someone cared about us.

The signs explaining where to go and what to do were clear, big, and abundant. We got a ticket, but the sign assured us that, as patients, there would be no charge for parking, and there wasn't.

On arrival, we generally felt that much care and thought had gone into arranging things for the benefit of the patients and making them feel special. In fact, employee parking was in a separate building distant from the hospital entrance. There was no question about it: Here, patients were special and more important than employees.

The heart center was on the sixth floor. Everything there was spick and span clean, and the place smelled good. The hallways and rooms were monochromatic white, with few pictures and no decorations. Mysterious blue signs hung on doors announcing that this was the door to a shelter room and that those who stayed there should remain quiet. That, I guess, was in case of an active shooter. In the old days, we never had active shooters, but now they have them in schools, 45 in 2024.

Two clerks greeted us, checked the computer, and showed us where to wait. There were no forms to fill out, no questions about who was going to pay, and no insurance check. This was a contrast with my previous experiences and made us feel welcome.

The waiting room had one other person, who was a hospital employee on break. On the large TV on the south wall, a program talked about houses that were difficult to sell and how to get the houses in better shape for sale. This was a stark contrast to Methodist Hospital, where the TV had an evangelical preacher with a bible in hand explaining something I don't know what because I muted the sound. At Methodist, another time, when I waited over an hour for the ultrasound of my liver (cost of scan $2,500), a TV had a video of a family reciting a prayer. That video played over and over, and there was no way to mute the sound.

Naturally, I complained, but the secretary couldn't do anything. She just shrugged her shoulders and said, "I just work here."

Sure enough, at noon on the dot, Ethel and I were ushered into the cardiac care room. A team of nurses sat at monitors in a high-tech setting that looked like it came right out of Star Wars. A nice, friendly nurse from Kenya introduced herself and hooked up the monitor, displaying Ethel's electrocardiogram, blood oxygen, pulse, respirations, and blood pressure. The nurse asked questions and told us what to expect and when to expect it. At least 20 minutes were spent, and all of Ethel's questions were answered, and a good history was taken of Ethel's general medical condition, medicines, allergies, and so forth.

I myself was deeply impressed with the humanity displayed by the staff and the time spent with us. They lifted a great burden of apprehension. Ethel and I are doctors, but we are still afraid of doctors and hospitals. I can only imagine what normal patients feel. We had no fear that decisions were being made behind our backs. Everything was open and above board. Why did we feel that way? Answer: Warm human contact. Nothing a hospital could provide in the way of technological marvels was as helpful as an atmosphere of compassion and friendly empathy.

The central question we ask about hospitals, and the question you should ask about hospitals and about doctors, for that matter, is whether you/we are in the right place. Does this place inspire confidence or not? Do we trust the place and the people to heal us? In short, can we expect good things will happen?

Ethel's cardiologist came in and shook our hands. Doctor Georg Carayannopoulos has been following Ethel for years. He knows her, and she knows him. Continuity of care was another big plus. He has a friendly face, a great smile, and excellent body language. He explained in detail what he was going to do, where he would make the small incision to get to the battery, and so forth. Questions were answered in detail, and consent forms were explained in detail and signed.

I was simply amazed that so much time was spent with us. Time with the doctor is what patients crave, and Doctor Carayannopoulos delivered. He explained that the operation itself would take about 32 minutes, but wheeling in and preparing the skin surface would take some time before, and applying the bandage would take time after. All in all, he told me I could expect that Ethel would return in about one hour.

Next, the anesthesiologist arrived. Same upbeat, happy attitude. He asked lots of questions and actually checked the anesthesia record from Ethel's cataract surgery many years ago. He introduced his assistant, David, who also had personality. It was decided to follow the previous anesthesia since it had worked well. Again, I was astounded that time had been taken to check a previous medical record and that the checking had resulted in what would likely be a riskless anesthesia.

They whisked Ethel away at 2:13, and she was back at 4 minutes to 3. Everything went well, and the doctors and nurses were obviously pleased and happy, and so were we.

And what to our wondering eyes should appear but a scientist/technician from Boston Scientific, the company that made Ethel's life-saving pacemaker. He explained things, answered questions, and gave Ethel an information book about the device.

Naturally, we were happy with him, the doctors, the nurses, the service, and with the result.

Total Bill: $43,000. Due from us—nothing.

AND AS FOR ME, I AM ELATED TO END THIS BOOK ON THAT HAP-PY NOTE.

THIS LAST ENCOUNTER PROVED IT WAS POSSIBLE TO PRACTICE MODERN MEDICINE WITH A HUMAN TOUCH.

FUTURE HEALTH CARE COULD BE AS GOOD AS WE GOT AT THE UNIVERSITY OF TEXAS MEDICAL BRANCH, GALVESTON.

HENCEFORTH, I CONTINUE TO HAVE A DISTINCT NOSTALGIA FOR THE PAST BUT ALSO A HOPE FOR THE POTENTIAL FUTURE OF MEDICINE THAT IS BOTH HUMANISTIC AND SCIENTIFIC.

THE READER MUST FORM HIS/HER OPINION ON THIS AS ON MANY OTHER MATTERS.

OFTEN, I LIE AWAKE AT NIGHT, STARING INTO THE BLACKNESS OF UNBORN TIME, WONDERING WHAT SHAPE THIS GREAT MEDICAL DRAMA WILL FINALLY TAKE AND WHERE THE SCENE OF THE NEXT ACT WILL BE LAID. I AM BY NATURE AN OPTIMIST, BUT FRANKLY THE UNBORN FUTURE DOESN'T LOOK THAT GREAT.

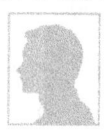

VALE:
FAREWELL AND GOODBYE

VALE: FAREWELL AND GOODBYE

◆ ◆ ◆

All good things have to come to an end. And this book is no exception. Sorry about that. Try to hold back your tears while I explain that where you go from here is entirely up to you. You can hang yourself. (Not advised) Or, you can just sit back and do nothing and continue to let them exploit you until you die and then, perhaps, you will get your eternal reward in heaven or some better place. Or, you can do something to improve the situation. You can even do something now. You can acquire more skill and knowledge and use your skill and knowledge to fight back. Yes. You can fight back. If you fight back, the odds are on your side. If you pussyfoot around the odds are not on your side and the system will continue to take you to the cleaners. It is up to you. You can try to be the master of your fate, the captain of your soul. Or you can let it ride. Spend some time thinking about your future directions. Meanwhile, I sincerely wish you ---

Good luck!

Your friend,

Bernie

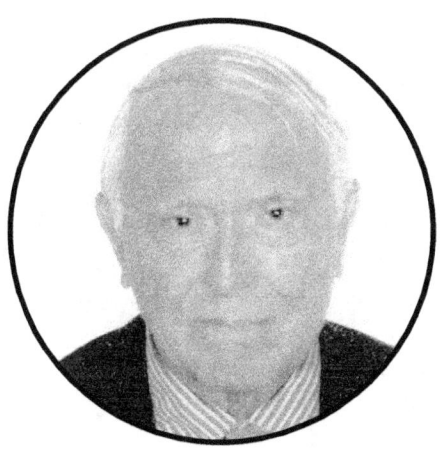

Suggested viewing:

The Rainmaker (1997).

This film covers most of the tricks the Great Benefits insurance company plays to get out of paying what they should have paid. The claim for a bone marrow transplant for acute myelogenous leukemia was denied, just the way every other claim made that year was denied. The corporate handbook, which they somehow got into evidence, explains every dirty trick to maximize profits by delay, denial, and ultimately, defending in court what they did. Of course, due to the law's delay, the kid dies before the treatment can be given. The jury sees through the corporate smokescreen and awards $50 million to the kid's estate. But Great Benefits goes through bankruptcy and in the end pays nothing.

The story, by attorney-turned-very-successful-author John Grisham, is quite interesting and realistic as well. The screenplay was written by, and the film was directed by Francis Ford Coppola. This film has wonderful courtroom drama and a great "legal world" introduction to the problems of proving intentional malfeasance, which is necessary for punitive damages.

The Road to Wellville (2020).

This movie, which I recommend as one of the major comedies of all time, shows how the promise of Health is the open sesame to the sucker's purse. Watch it and you will laugh your head off. It tells of the famous San and the kind of zany people who visited it for " the cure " of their bowels or the Green Disease or their neuroses or whatever. There is some exaggeration for the fun of it, but basically the film gives a realistic impression of what the San were like in the 1880s and what happened there. Anthony Hopkins once again proves his acting ability as the infamous Dr Kellogg, the director of the San. His recipe for success is a 15-gallon daily enema followed by yogurt, by mouth and per rectum. "With a friend like him, who needs an enema?" says one of the patients. While prescribing enemas for his patients daily, Doctor Kellogg saw sex as the killer that hastens the death of both men and women. Hence, sex at the San was prohibited, a no-no. But, despite the good doctor's prohibition, that no-no never works for long in the movie or for that matter in life itself. After you watch the movie, read the book, which is more historically accurate and even more fun.

Suggested Reading:

The Road to Wellville by T.C. Boyle. Penguin Books, 1993.

This is one of my all-time favorite books. The story is fascinating, and the writing is extraordinary. Boyle is able to describe things with such detail and accuracy that it truly comes alive on the page. He has a wild sense of humor, and if you are open to it, there are spots where you will literally put down the book and laugh. Many lessons are taught by Boyle's detailed historical scholarship, but the main one in my view is we contemporary people are just as susceptible to health bullshit as people were in the 1880s and early 1990s. Promote a scheme to give a promise of health and longevity, and you will get rich quick.

Making Them Pay: How to Get the Most from Health Insurance and Managed Care by Rhonda D. Orin. St. Martin's Griffin Press, 2001.

Rhonda is a lawyer with lots of experience suing insurance companies on behalf of policyholders and herself, fighting for the kids in her own family. Most people don't understand insurance, and the insurance companies know it. They use their advantage to perpetrate unfair denials, late payments, and hopeless confusion. This gem of a book gives lots of great advice on how to get around the obstructions and smokescreens and get what you deserve to be paid. The cartoons are an excellent way of breaking up what can be a boring subject and helping us develop the proper mental attitude to fight for our rights as patients.

Making them pay has two cardinal virtues: it's practical and funny. For Rhonda Orin, fighting a health insurer over a coverage denial or a short payment seems to be like fox-hunting for an English nobleman: a joy to be studied with relish and pursued at every opportunity. Recalcitrance or feigned incompetence on the part of an insurer only stimulates her to fight harder -- and this book spells out how to make the companies suffer. Here we also have a somewhat dated guide to choosing an insurance plan, if you're lucky enough to have a choice, and to reading the policy with an eye to hidden costs and hidden exclusions. Mrs. Orin writes about insurers as if they're incorrigible children -- children she knows need discipline.

Your insurance company doesn't want you to read this book. So, go ahead and read it.

DELAY DENY DEFEND: Why Insurance Companies Don't Pay Claims And What You Can Do About It by Jay M. Feinman.

Delay, Deny, Defend offers a compelling deep dive into the realities of dealing with the insurance industry, shedding light on the complex and often frustrating processes behind claims. The book brilliantly illustrates a range of cases—spanning health insurance, car accidents, and property coverage—and tracks how these systems, initially designed for protection and support, have shifted into mechanisms that often prioritize profit over fairness.

Feinman, a professor of law, unpacks the tactics many insurance companies use: delaying claim responses, denying valid claims, and aggressively defending their decisions in legal battles. He provides readers with essential insights into how to navigate these challenges effectively. The book doesn't sugarcoat the reality—it makes clear that fighting against these tactics can be a long and arduous process.

There came a time 20 or so years ago when, like the banking industry, the insurance industry sold its soul to the devil of profit. This book is the classic that explains how the industry has employed top consultancies to devise strategies to ensure that the consumer making an insurance claim gets paid as little as possible, or better still, not at all. The title delay, deny, defend is one of those strategies. Another is to pay a fortune in advertising to create the myth that your insurance company will be there for you when you need them. Very often, they won't. They are not your friend. Their sole objective is to maximize profits for their shareholders and maximize the pay of their senior executives.... no matter what human misery they cause along the way.

Overall, Delay, Deny, Defend is an eye-opening read that serves as both a warning and a guide. It highlights the necessity of understanding the system and approaching it with clear eyes, even if it doesn't offer a definitive resolution to the broader industry problems.

Claims Game: The Deceptive Tactics Insurance Companies Use To Underpay Or Deny Your Claim by David Skipton. Lulu Publishing (2015).

Excellent discussion of the tricks and how to get around them. Time and energy are needed to defeat the enemy but often you can win. This gem of a book covers mainly the claims that arise from property damage. I loved the way David explained how the companies handle the slab cases. A storm rushes through, and people return to find only a slab of their home remains. Insurance will claim the destruction was caused by whatever is not covered and ask you to prove differently. Some states have already handled this problem by imposing the burden of proof on the companies and not on you. The major message is again that insurance companies once looked out for customers, but not now. You need to know what motivates them if you want any chance of collecting what you are owed.

Example: If a hail storm damages your windshield, is that functional or cosmetic damage? Is it covered? Companies have often argued cosmetic damage is excluded. If that were true, they would have a hard time selling auto insurance and there would be millions of autos out there looking like they have been in a demolition derby. The whole idea of purchasing insurance is to protect your property from damage, functional or cosmetic, it doesn't matter. If you don't fight, they will win. If you do fight, the odds are way on your side, and the chances are you will win.

And Finally: Matters of Life and Death by Henry Marsh. St. Martin's Press (2022).

Marsh tells what it is like for a mature, respected physician to become a patient, experiencing words and deeds intended to bring solace, but having a completely different effect because he is a doctor and knows the ropes and what's what and why. In my view, basically, he doesn't like being a patient, he doesn't like getting old, he doesn't like the aches and pains in his joints, and he doesn't like his failing vision, and he doesn't like having prostate cancer. Who would? He doesn't like the medicine he takes for his prostate cancer that tends to castrate him, and he doesn't like the doctors and some of the nurses and the technicians. He wants to be treated with more tenderness. But actually, the National Health Service, which some people have proposed as the role model for American National health insurance, worked pretty well. Because it works so well, Marsh just has health problems to worry about and not insurance problems. That is a significant benefit when you are sick, and something which we Americans should think about.

Taste of my own medicine: When the doctor is the patient by Dr. Edward E. Rosenbaum. Random House (1988)

Nothing unusual about a patient venting spleen at the doctor, but in this instance the patient is a doctor. And with his forceful, angry book, Ed establishes himself as a "patient advocate," for during his own medical treatment, a rheumatologist Rosenbaum (now dead) says he "learned more about handling the seriously ill . . . than in 50 years of practice."

Rosenbaum, suffering with cancer of the larynx, kept a journal during his therapy. He records his threats to bring a malpractice suit against the doctors who misdiagnosed his affliction for nine months, because, according to him, they used the wrong equipment to look at his throat. He rails against the indifference and incompetence of those administering his X-ray treatments and expresses his resentment at the radiotherapist's lack of compassion.

Rosenbaum has strong opinions as well about medicine's turn toward big business techniques, the profit motive, and cost-effectiveness; he criticizes insurance carriers, Medicare and Medicaid.

His rancor should have been a bitter pill to the brethren. But time has marched on. The treatments have become more effective for some diseases, but the human touch has by and large not improved, and the big business effect on medical care is worse than ever.

The Great American Medicine Show: Being an Illustrated History of HUCKSTERS, HEALERS, Health Evangelists, and HEROES from Plymouth Rock to the PRESENT by David Armstrong and Elizabeth Metzger Armstrong. Printice Hall (1991).

This is a well-written and well-researched disquisition of the various items mentioned in the title and subtitle. The weird use of capitals and italics is the publisher's and authors', not mine.

The index and bibliography notes are excellent. Spotlighted are the bizarre and bold, the stupid and the absolutely crazy health gimmicks of America's past and recent present. Read here about crusaders and reformers, crackpots and quacks who are as American as apple pie. Attacked are herbalism, homeopathy, temperance, hydrotherapy, phrenology, patent medicines, evangelism. Fletcherizing, chiropractic, physical culture, fad diets, and exercise crazes. Many of the off-the-wall cures and treatments are lavishly illustrated with vintage photographs. Read and laugh and, also, read and weep. Oh America! How I mourn for you that you are so gullible. It is really puzzling to me how this magnificent masterpiece of scholarship is not well distributed and well read. Alas, real scholarship in America is seldom appreciated or rewarded, and often must labor uphill.

FINISH.

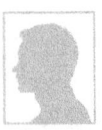

APPENDIX

APPENDIX

◆ ◆ ◆

No Explanation Necessary

By Allegra Patten, MD

The sixtieth birthday party of a medical school classmate was a great time to catch up with friends. They know I am now happily working as a substitute teacher, despite training to be a neurologist. When I talk to other doctors who are friends of friends, I try to think of how to sum up the reason for a career change. How do I do it succinctly over a cocktail?

The reason is not any of the difficult parts of medicine that I knew about from the beginning. We knew what we signed up for. I knew the job could be risky and messy, especially in medical school, when I accidentally overlooked the respiratory precautions sign on the room of a veteran with tuberculosis and spent an hour talking to him without a mask. The nursing staff was appalled and really worried about me. During internship training, when the needle covers changed on the "safety syringes' to something unfamiliar, I accidentally stuck myself with a needle from an HIV positive, Hepatitis C-positive patient. Luckily, I did not get those diseases. In residency, a demented patient urinated on me. In addition, there were times when I had to examine prisoners who came with guards. These things I expected.

The 112-hour work week in the internship made the hours in practice a comparative relief. I knew there would be a night call. Most of my career, it was every other night or every third. The transfer center would sometimes wake me at 2 AM to tell me about a patient that they **might** need me to accept. They weren't sure if the hospital had beds, but they would call me back if beds were available, probably around 3 AM. Some patients called at night because it was convenient. One wanted a refill at two in the morning. He worked the night shift. Driving to see a stroke patient on New Year's Eve just after midnight, hoping I wouldn't run across a drunk driver on my path, was part of the job.

I also knew that working with the public can be difficult. People were sometimes angry when I explained how I avoid prescribing narcotics. My spiel about how narcotics can actually trigger chronic headaches was met with an embarrassingly loud, "This doctor is a crock of shit," as one drug seeker headed out to the waiting room. In addition, I had to "fire" a patient for lying to me. He assured me that he had a driver to take him home after I gave him a strong injectable headache medication that would impair driving. He had planned to drive himself, despite the danger to others on the road. One time, I even had to talk to a patient about treating my Black secretary with respect, or I could not be their physician. On another occasion, I had no choice but to transfer a patient back to their referring hospital, because they refused care from a woman doctor. I was the only neurologist in the hospital over the weekend. By far, the most difficult interactions were telling someone or their family that they would be permanently blind, or paralyzed, or brain-dead.

Next, there were things I didn't like that I hadn't been prepared for in training. Students don't get to observe attending physicians spending one hour trying to get a test that is clearly medically necessary, approved by an insurance company. I never got a denial when I went through the motions. I always did these prior approvals for my patients, despite no compensation, other than the relief of the patient when I told them, "I got it approved." But I really needed to be at daycare after clinic, not doing this.

Then came the electronic medical record, the EMR. Before it, I used to clear all my charts at the end of a day, dictating summaries of the patients' care to their referring physician, calling patients with lab results, and reviewing records. After our practice adopted the electronic medical record, my afternoon "off" was now spent trying to check boxes and figure out how to enter things, so they would actually be what I had really done. If I checked that a patient had normal strength in their shins, the program would print out that I had had the patient walk on their heels. But I had tested shin strength in a different way.

Dictating summaries was phased out, and the physician had to do all the typing. Thank God for Ms. Holmquist, my eighth-grade typing teacher. Ironically, I remember my classmates saying, "Allegra, why are you taking typing? You're not going to be a secretary." Because the EMR was such a pain, some doctors cut and pasted prior summaries they had typed. That meant when I reviewed charts, I was rereading information, wasting more time.

I also didn't figure that my salary would drop as the years went on. Malpractice premiums soared, even though I had no claims against me. I had read that one-third of physicians do have to deal with being sued. Reimbursement went down, not keeping up with inflation. By 2012, I was making $40,000 a year to work more than full-time, with nine years of training beyond college and 20 years of experience in my field.

Ancillary help became less and less. If I wanted the ophthalmoscope fixed, they had to call someone off-site, which might take a week. Previously, the hospital handyman used to come in with a light bulb within the hour. I suspect that patient payments are now going towards medical administrators and insurance company employees, so hospitals and medical practices must cut staff members who really help deliver the care. And, why pay an employee to change the sheets between patients in the EMG lab, when the doctor can do that?

It came down to less and less time doing what I wanted to do, which was listening to patients and solving their problems. My **thing** was second and third opinions. No one pays for you to review stacks of records and really figure out someone's symptoms. I was ok not getting paid extra for that, but I no longer had the time to do it. I was too busy talking to insurance companies, typing, getting a light bulb, and changing the sheets.

I wasn't surprised when I thought about all the women doctors at this birthday party and how their initial paths had changed. Lana wasn't happy, but didn't know what to do about it. Misha called radiology in Nashville, "a shit show." Mae was retiring early. Two women were doing concierge medicine to be able to spend more time with patients and make a decent living. Sela had quit OBGYN practice and was doing clinical research. Jana is now working as a pilot. "Flying to make is living is more fun than medicine, "she said. And I am now a substitute teacher for elementary schools, no explanation necessary, if you are talking to other doctors.

Healthcare Is Sick

By Tad Yoneyama, M.D.

The best analogy for the current state of healthcare that I can give is that US healthcare is in the ICU on life support. Based on my experience of over 30 years as a general practice doctor, I do not feel that there is any hope of recovery and recommend DNR—Do Not Resuscitate. The system is broken and we are beyond the point of no return.

In 2025, consumers (YOU) pay money to a health insurance company, then:

- They dictate which pharmacy you can use (and profit from it, check GoodRx.com for prices with and without insurance),
- They have set up companies to approve or decline authorization for radiology tests and share in the savings from declined tests that the doctor has deemed medically necessary (see MedSolutions/Evicore),
- Several major health insurance companies have settled lawsuits where they used software and policies to systematically decrease payments for services rendered by physicians.

A September 2024 article in JAMA (Journal of the American Medical Association) estimates that a primary care physician spends 7.3 hours in the EHR (electronic health record) for every 8 hours in the clinic seeing patients. So for every day seeing patients, doctors are having to work into the late night, weekends, holidays, and vacations.

I am humbled and honored by the privilege that my patients have allowed me to be a part of their family's health and wish that we could go back in time to the barter system that my grandfather was under when he was a family doctor. Unfortunately, I do not see the healthcare system changing, and see this as a terminal illness. I wish that I had the skills to fix it, but sadly do not.

www.ingramcontent.com/pod-product-compliance
Lightning Source LLC
Chambersburg PA
CBHW071716120626
46550CB00001B/259